Touchstones

Manual for the Crystal Therapist

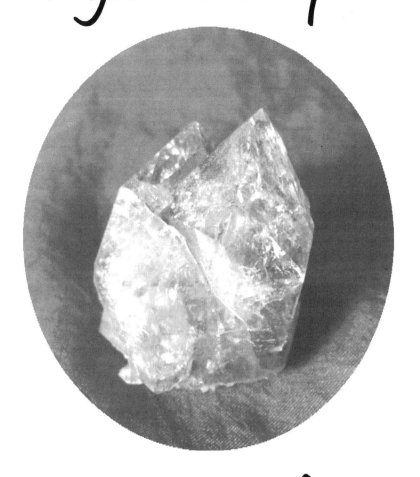

Lauren D'Silva

Touchstones: Manual for the Crystal Therapist
Black and White Edition
Lauren D'Silva

First edition published United Kingdom 2013
Second Edition published United Kingdom 2015

Touchstones School of Crystal Therapy
Llandrindod Wells
Powys UK
LD1 5NB

Disclaimer
        The information in this book is not intended as an alternative to seeking medical treatment, nor can it be used for diagnosis. You should consult a qualified physician if you have any concerns about your health. This manual was written to accompany a teacher led training course. If you are attempting to learn about Crystal Therapy by yourself and need assistance you should seek out a suitably qualified practitioner or teacher.
        You should not use this book without the prior approval of your Doctor if you are undergoing medical treatment or have any health issues, whether they be physical, emotional or mental. Pregnant women should seek medical advice. Neither the author nor the publisher will accept any liability for your health and wellbeing when using the exercises or information contained in this book.

Acknowledgements

My gratitude to all of my crystal teachers and mentors over the last 15 years. To Pam, my mother's yoga teacher and the therapist who gave me my first taste of the power of crystals. To Cassie, my original teacher, who gave me an excellent grounding in crystal work and fuelled my enthusiasm to learn more. To Elizabeth Goodacre with whom I studied for my SVA Diploma. To Nessa McHugh with whom I set up my first crystal healing business. To the Principals of ICGT, Sue and Simon Lilly, who welcomed us into their fold as their Tutors and who gave us the firm foundations we needed in the early days to deliver a Crystal Therapy Diploma course. To my ACHO Colleagues who welcomed me and my school into their fellowship and who have supported me as the Chair of the Affiliation of Crystal Healing Organisations.

My sincere thanks to my husband Steve for all his help and support over the years, for his help with the editing process and being the 'male body' in photos. Thanks also to Semele Xerri, the female 'body' for this manual and the photographer for my author photo. Finally thanks to the crystals themselves who are the best teachers I could ever ask for and from whom I am continually learning.

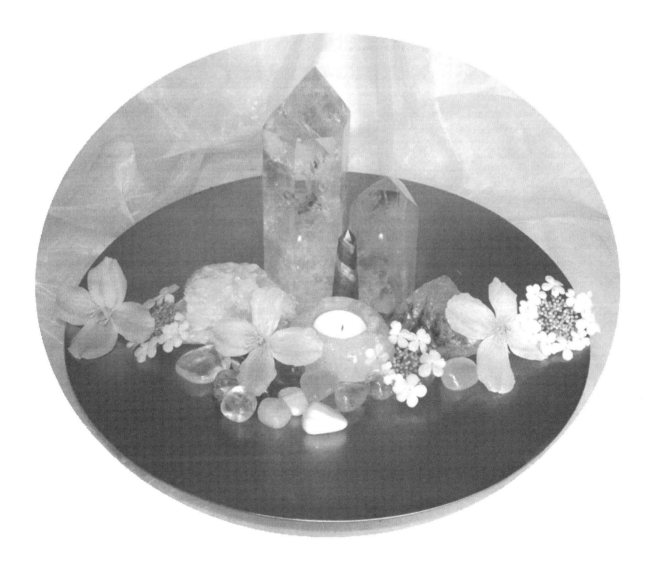

Contents

Foreword - Michael Eastwood

We live in an age where humanity is unfolding at a remarkable rate. For crystal healers the time is ripe to step forwards to assist in this process. This is the ideal book to assist on our continuing journey to wholeness.

What Lauren presents here arises from deep within her Being. Through her wise, clear guidance we are taken deep into the heart of the mineral kingdom. Our horizons are expanded as well as being nourished on so many levels.

Lauren's book is suitable for the experienced healer as well as those starting on the journey. This book takes us step by step and lesson by lesson through all that is needed to ground crystal intuition into a workable reality. It not only engages the reader through the exercises, but continually expands the reader's horizons as to what is possible. This book is rich in practical exercises that take the reader through everything one could need to become familiar with crystal healing.

We are gently guided into the crystal kingdom where we become familiar with many aspects of crystal healing; especially how to apply crystals in healing. We are encouraged to understand and work with the chakra system as well as the aura, which is usually a complex subject, yet in Lauren's writing all unfolds, grounded in simplicity.

Subjects such as choosing crystals, the holistic spine, healing from an eastern perspective, crystallography and advice for the crystal therapist are covered in Lauren's gentle yet clear writing style.

Touchstones is imbued with an unusual degree of insight and wisdom. For me, it is as though the mineral kingdom is itself expressing itself through this luminous book. I could not recommend this wonderful book and Lauren's crystal offerings through her teaching and healing work highly enough.

Michael is an international teacher of crystal healing with 25 years experience. He is the author of the best selling *The Crystal Oversoul Attunements* as well as *Unfolding Our Light* both published by Findhorn Press. He is also the co- writer of Prediction magazine's monthly articles on Crystal Healing - along with Margaret Ann Lembo. His ACHO credited teaching school the School of Soul Medicine has been teaching two year and post graduate diplomas in crystal healing for many years. He served as a former Chair of ACHO.

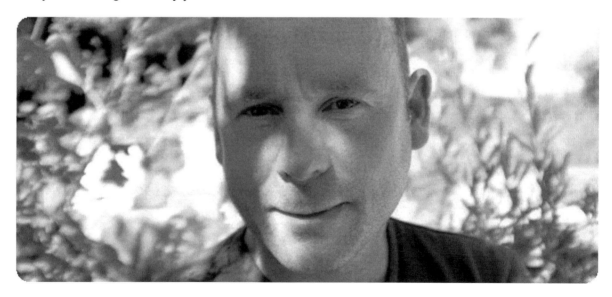

Using this Manual

This Manual was written primarily to support the Foundation and Certificate courses from Touchstones School of Crystal Therapy which between them cover the Affiliation of Crystal Healing Organisations (ACHO) Core Curriculum. If you intend to become a Crystal Therapist I strongly advise you to seek out a professional, thorough, training course as nothing beats learning from an experienced and capable teacher. Do not be tempted by 'qualify in a weekend', or 'qualify by correspondence' courses, they are simply not sufficient to work professionally in this field. Contact details for Touchstones School of Crystal Therapy and the Affiliation of Crystal Healing Organisations are given at the end of the book.

Please note that whilst Crystal Therapy is non-invasive and is considered to be a very safe form of therapy some people do have strong reactions. You can read more about Healing Crises in the chapter on Advice for the Crystal Therapist. Clients in a compromised state of health should seek medical advice before having Crystal Healing. You should not try to treat anyone beyond your level of experience as a therapist. Crystal Therapy may be contraindicated for people with mental health issues and addictions, particularly for the inexperienced therapist. Women in the first trimester of pregnancy should avoid Crystal Therapy. Children and the elderly may also require treatment from someone with more experience.

Do use the techniques described here for your own wellbeing so that you understand how it feels to receive a crystal treatment. It is always more fun if you can team up with a willing friend and learn together. Keep a Journal to record your progress.

Some pages are marked 'Photocopy friendly' and are included to help you keep records and make useful charts that you can write on or laminate.

What is a Touchstone?

Historically a touchstone was a hard black stone used to test the quality of precious metals such as gold and silver according to the colour streak they made when scratched upon it. Now the term is more often used metaphorically as a sign of validity and quality. I see a touchstone as something that is enduring and dependable in the way that crystals and stones are. For me touchstones bring you back into connection with your eternal essence, your true Self.

In this manual the Touchstones are my suggested crystals for each topic. They are not intended as an exhaustive list, so if you are drawn to use something else please do so. My descriptions of the crystal properties are borne out of personal experience. These findings cannot be scientifically proven, not yet at least, I am simply imparting what I feel about the stones and how I have observed their energies.

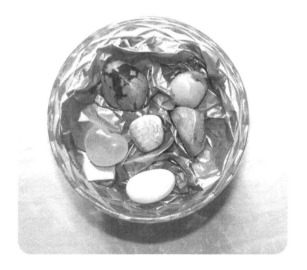

Keeping a Personal Development Journal: Know Thyself

Successful, effective healers have got a good understanding of what makes them tick. They will have been willing to work through their major issues and are aware of their foibles and idiosyncrasies. You don't need to be 'perfect' to be a therapist, but you do need to be self aware and self reflective. Make a commitment to yourself to unfold, develop and grow as you walk your healing path.

A personal development journal can help you to explore and understand the synchronicities, opportunities and challenges that come your way as you walk your spiritual path. Kept well, it will record your experiences and provide you with a place to jot down ideas, messages, or inspiration as you receive it. If you are studying an ACHO course then keeping your journal is a course requirement.

Any notebook can become your personal development journal, but to encourage you to revisit and write entries I suggest treating yourself to a really special journal. I have a stack of journals filled over the years and I like to look back at them from time to time and reflect on insights and experiences that I might otherwise have forgotten.

You may record anything you feel is significant in your journal, for example:

Impressions or sensations you have had whilst healing or being healed
Sensations, images, or messages received during meditations
Dreams
Moments of synchronicity
Intuitive experiences
Interesting information from workshops you've attended
Quotations that touch you
Sketches of images seen in your third eye
Reflections on your spiritual path
Key points from books you have read
Photos or drawings of your latest crystal purchases with notes about them
Questions you want to raise with your teacher or research further

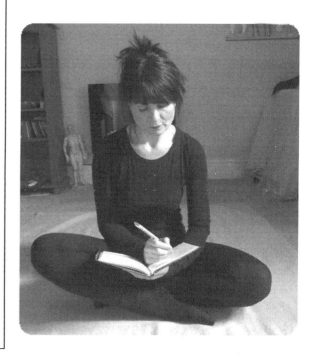

Your journal should be something you feel tempted to turn back to and read again, so make it as lovely as you like. Often when you look back at your journal you will get an 'Aha!' moment, as pieces of a puzzle slip into place, or you notice new connections or patterns. Do keep a journal; you will find it is a tool for reflection and self development, as well as a fascinating document recording your journey.

When I was going through the period of my life documented in my past life autobiographical story 'Light Behind the Angels' I kept copious notes. Without my journals I wouldn't have been able to write the book. Time and again I would return to my notebooks and find episodes recorded that I'd forgotten about, but that made sense in light of later events. You never know how useful a journal may be to you!

Chapter One:
How do Crystals Work?

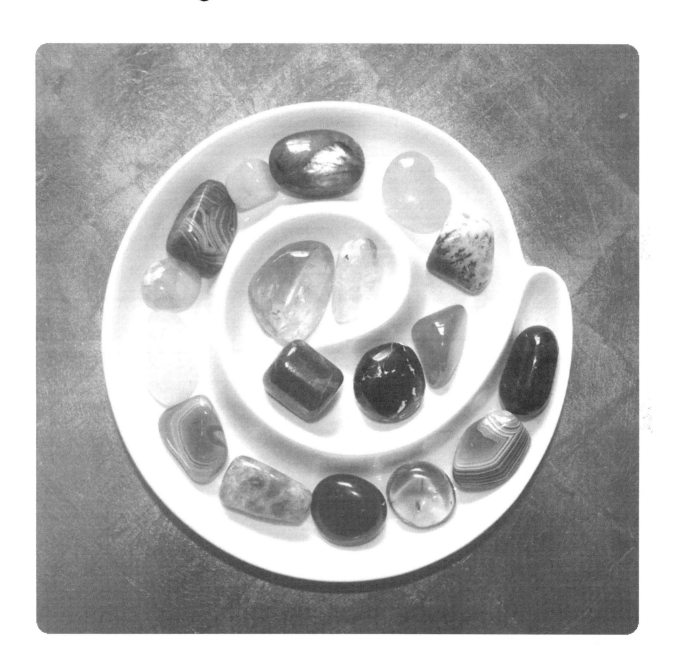

How Does Crystal Healing Work?

As a crystal therapist I am often asked how crystals 'work'. The simple answer is no-one is absolutely sure, but in my experience they do! We are yet to come up with a definitive explanation, but we do have some theories and beliefs about the way crystals bring about therapeutic changes for people.

Let's look at some of the more scientific explanations. The most helpful theory comes from the world of quantum physics. Quantum physicists have proven that everything in the Universe is made of energy and that energy is in a constant state of vibration. Even apparently solid inanimate objects are formed of moving energy at the subatomic level. If you took an electron microscope and looked into anything, however solid to the naked eye, you would find lots of space within, much more space than matter.

Because of their orderly crystalline lattice structure crystals are very good at holding a constant and stable vibration. Many crystals can remain essentially unchanged over tens of thousands, even millions, of years. We, on the other hand, are an incredibly complex and dynamically changing mix of vibrations and our energies can get easily disturbed and go out of balance, which can cause illness. Our bodies constantly need to discard and replace cells and eventually we physically decline. Even the healthiest individual has a lifespan that is infinitesimal compared to our crystalline friends. Lots of things can affect our energy, from external influences such as electromagnetic and geopathic stress, to internal ones such as poor diet, constant negative thought patterns and suppressing emotions.

Quantum physics states that everything is interconnected, however separated and individual we imagine ourselves to be. You cannot change one thing without subtly affecting everything else. When a crystal therapist places crystals on or around a client they are intending to find the right healing vibrations for the client. When crystals are well chosen their steady vibrations encourage the parts of the body experiencing discord to realign their own vibrations and return to harmony.

One way to explain this process to the layman is to use the analogy of a large symphony orchestra. When all the instruments are in tune and the players are playing the right notes at the right time the overall sound produced is a delight to listen to. When one instrument goes out of tune the small notes of discord may not be immediately noticeable, however musicians sitting around that player soon become distracted and also start to play off key. Soon the disharmony spreads and the music becomes a cacophony. The instrument that caused the discord needs retuning and the player needs to play in time with the rest of the orchestra. So it is with our bodies. We are made of many complex systems, such as our digestive system, nervous system and cardiovascular system. Our systems have multiple components that need to work together harmoniously for our overall good health. When one part of our physiology falters and starts to 'play out of tune' we may not notice much at first, but if the balance is not restored then other parts of our system can be affected and we experience ill health. The application of crystals can be thought of like a tuning fork for the body, restoring the correct vibrations and so bringing back harmony to the whole system.

Crystal therapy can also be explained using colour theory. White light can be refracted into the spectrum of rainbow colours. This is what happens when sunlight shines through raindrops and creates a rainbow. Each colour has its own specific vibrational frequency and wavelength, each of which have an effect on health. The application of coloured light is already a medically accepted tool for healing certain conditions, such as jaundice in newborn babies. Colour therapists are aware that colour has wider ranging applications and colour is an effective therapy in its own right. Crystals come in a wide range of colours and different crystals of a similar colour will share some key healing properties. Each crystal can be regarded as carrying a frequency of light in a stable form easily applied to the client. Clear quartz and other transparent crystals can be viewed as like working with white light, carrying the full spectrum within themselves, which is one reason that clear quartz is often regarded as a master healer.

Another scientific theory is based on crystalline structures. Although there are thousands of different crystals, there are just seven crystal structures. Sometimes we can see the structure externally in the shape of the crystal, for example in the six sided, hexagonal structure of beryls, such as aquamarine and emerald, or the cubic structure of iron pyrites or fluorite, which sometimes form literally as cubes. More often the structure is internal and not so obvious to the eye, but it exists in a tumble stone just as much as in a perfect crystal specimen. There are several theories about how the seven different structures of crystals can be related to healing. Some therapists link the seven structures to the seven main chakras. Michael Gienger has probably evolved the most intriguing theory. He has observed that just as there are seven structures in crystals there are seven corresponding personality types in humans and we all have a dominant one. He then applies the crystals on a 'like heals like basis' similar to homeopathy.

Many crystal therapists are more comfortable connecting with their crystals in an esoteric rather than a scientific way. Think of this. Crystals come from the Earth and help connect us back to our Earth Mother. In modern times we tend to live lives that seem rather removed from Nature and connecting with these beautiful stones can remind us that we are also part of the natural world. Some think that our disconnection from the rhythms and energies of Nature is the underlying cause of many of our ailments, whether they be physical, emotional, mental or spiritual.

Crystals are often truly ancient. They are stable and enduring whereas our lives are full of turmoil and fleeting in comparison. Our Spirit however is eternal and many crystal therapists believe we are reborn many times. Holding a crystal can remind us of our true eternal nature and steady us through the changing fortunes of our lives. Crystals can also link us to ancient times and ancient wisdom. Healers are often drawn to healing with crystals because they have done so before. For many of us this method of healing is more of a remembering than a new field of learning.

Although modern man may view crystals as 'lifeless lumps of rock' traditional peoples saw them as having their own form of consciousness. Native Americans refer to crystals as the 'Stone people'. Shamanic journeying and meditations with crystals are perhaps the easiest ways to make a connection. Often your stones have wisdom to convey, so please be respectful, you are a visitor to their world. Because crystals don't run around with 'to do' lists they never get distracted from, or lose contact with their inner wisdom. Some people channel knowledge from their crystals and use that insight to guide them. Rather than seeing crystals as simply tools to be used, healers who work in this way are moving into a relationship of co-creation with their stones.

So whether you are a dyed in the wool scientist, or a mystic, you can see that there are many possible ways that crystals can bring about a healing response. From years of experience I know crystal healing works beyond any reasonable doubt and I look forward to the day that crystal therapy is accepted in more mainstream settings.

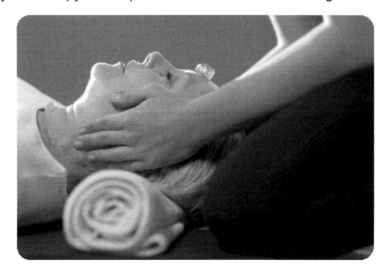

The New Science: Quantum Physics

Whilst Crystal Therapy can be viewed as a highly intuitive art, it is becoming clear that there may be a sound scientific basis to the way in which it and other energy therapies work. For some this is reassuring and validates the therapy while others may prefer an air of magic and mystery! I feel that it is good to be able to explain your therapy work in more scientific terms as far as you are able to and that the new science that does explain this is quite magical in its own right.

Orthodox medicine largely follows a cause and effect model of reality. From this point of view the human body is a complex machine controlled by the brain and peripheral nervous system, which today's doctors might compare to a powerful on-board computer. Surgical approaches may patch up, replace, or remove worn out or malfunctioning parts. Drug based approaches introduce substances to the body to correct a lack, or a malfunction, or to fight an invading organism in the case of antibiotics for example. These methods are very successful for some health issues. Hip replacements, for example, have made many people's lives much more comfortable and antibiotics can be a real life saver.

What's Missing in this Model?

Orthodox medicine has some clear weaknesses. Two people of very similar constitution won't necessarily react the same way to a drug treatment for example. Side effects from the same drugs vary enormously between people. Doctors and drug companies can only report the range of side effects possible, prediction for an individual is not usually possible or accurate. If we are so mechanistic in our design why are we so variable in our responses? Orthodox medicine is unable to account for the reason one person's tumour will progress quickly and prove fatal, whereas another person with a similar tumour will go into remission and make a good recovery. If we were like physical machines you might reasonably expect us to be more predictable in our health.

Quantum Physics

In the 20th Century Quantum Physicists proved beyond doubt that all matter is comprised of energy. Everything in existence is in a constant state of movement or vibration. Atoms are not inert beads, as they are represented in school chemistry sets; they are like tiny whirling solar systems.

Humans are made of complex energy fields. Pharmacological and surgical approaches to healing ignore the vital forces which animate and breathe life into the biomachinery of living systems. A Quantum Physicist's view of vibrational medicine might express the human being as a multidimensional organism made up of complex energy fields in dynamic interplay with each other. Vibrational healing such as crystal therapy works on the subtle energy fields of the body. Using crystals we can 'fine tune' these energetic systems to resonate in greater harmony and promote health.

Key Ideas to Grasp from Quantum Physics

Quantum physics is still in its infancy, but it is bringing us new ways of understanding the Universe which are often strikingly similar to the ways that mystics and Shamen have envisioned the Universe for millennia. Some of these ideas have such huge and mind blowing implications for how we choose to live our lives that we revert to a comfortable mechanical world view because it is easier to think about the world that way!

Here are some of the ideas and theories coming through from the world of quantum physics which I feel have exciting implications for us as healers. Just imagine the possibilities!

Most of matter is empty space.

Matter is like an energetic wave with infinite potential, it is only when we observe it that it becomes particulate and fixed, therefore our perceptions create our reality.

We only process a minute fraction of the information which surrounds us all of the time.

Changing your focus will change your reality.

All realities may exist simultaneously. Linear time is an artificial construct.

Our minds create our bodies.

At a subatomic level we are One unified energy field. The thought and energy patterns we each emit go out into the Field and so influence the Whole.

Chapter Two:
Care for your Energy

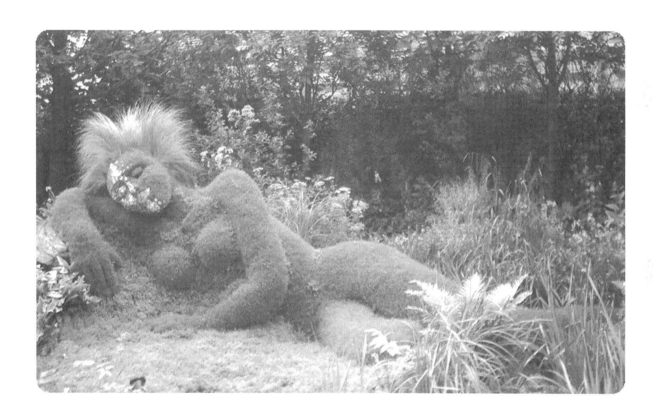

Are You a Healer?

To a certain extent anyone can heal and most people at some time in their lives will have unconsciously given healing. It is the kind of energy a mother naturally passes to her sick child as she holds him, or a lover uses to comfort a grieving partner. Anyone can be trained to choose a crystal and place it to precipitate a healing response, therefore you don't have to be a natural healer to work with crystals therapeutically.

Healers carry the need to give healing as part of their life purpose. Many have already been drawn to caring professions such as nursing, or to other complementary therapies. Healers can actually become unwell themselves if they block their abilities and don't allow the healing energy to flow. A healer does not require an 'attunement' to be able to transfer healing energy, although some choose to have these done.

So how can you tell? You may be told of your ability. When I look at someone I 'know' if they are a healer. Ask yourself, when you see a hurt child, or someone who is ill or upset, do your hands tingle or your palms buzz? Maybe you sense warmth in your hands? This is the result of the minor chakras becoming activated in your palms so that healing energy can flow out through them. Healing energy may leave the palms speckled and mottled as it passes through, turning the hands pinker too, so take a look next time this happens! People may comment on how warm your hands feel to them. Maybe your heart chakra opens automatically when you hear a baby cry and you feel warmth in the centre of your chest? Perhaps you just know what to do to bring comfort to another person, or you are the one everyone brings their problems to and people say they feel better when they've spoken to you.

Some other experiences that healers tend to have before they learn to channel the energy include receiving lots of static shocks. Car doors always used to get me before I started healing! This I believe is a discharge of built up energy in the healer's hands; it improves once you start using the energy. I've also had bizarre effects on electrical items and gave up on wearing watches as they never lasted long. I think this was due to a build-up of energy in my aura. Since using my healing gift I rarely have these difficulties, although I still prefer not to wear a wristwatch.

Healers tend to be empathic. Many have auras that soak up feelings from others like sponges. You may find that you pick up someone else's stomach-ache, headache, or depressed mood for example. If this is happening pay particular attention to the protection of your aura. It needs to be resilient enough for everyday life. It isn't comfortable to be so sensitive all the time, although it may be useful when you need to understand how another person is feeling. As a therapist you need clear enough boundaries to work out what is your 'stuff' and what is someone else's.

Natural healers do benefit from giving healing, whether professionally or to their nearest and dearest, so that the healing energy is running freely and not blocked up. A client of mine knew he was a healer but didn't do any healing because he felt 'tired all the time'. He was worried that giving healing would drain him further. However by giving healing little and often his own energy levels improved somewhat. If you think of healing energy as if it is water running through a pipe then this is not surprising. In the act of conducting the water the pipe is kept free flowing. If it can't flow the water stagnates. In the same way healing energy passes through us, keeping us clear to channel more good energy.

Healers must always be aware that they are allowing universal healing energy to flow through themselves, not giving their own life force energy away. A shaman would refer to this as being like a hollow bone; it is the art of getting your ego out of the way so that the energy can flow unhindered. Always ensure you are well grounded before you begin any sort of healing. Grounding prevents excess energy building in your system so please read the section on grounding carefully.

Listening to the Still Small Voice Within

We are always connected to our Higher Self, which some regard as the incorruptible essence of the soul which is connected to the Divine. It is to the Higher Self that we connect when healing, as here we can contact true wisdom free from our Ego self's judgements and opinions. Be aware that this 'inner voice' can seem small and quiet compared to our normal waking thoughts. This is why practices such as meditation are recommended to help you become more aware of your own guidance; when you are sitting still your mind is more receptive and can become quiet enough to listen within.

Our onboard guidance mechanism is best described as intuition, literally 'tuition from within' or a kind of inner knowing. The more we listen to our intuition the stronger it becomes, a bit like exercising a spiritual muscle! Following our intuition can reap huge rewards in life and prevent some unnecessary struggles too. My own inner voice has literally been a life-saver. By listening to and following your intuition you are placing your trust in the wiser aspect of your Self and you can more easily 'go with the flow'. This doesn't excuse you from taking necessary actions or doing any work of course!

Personal development work, in particular journal keeping, recording of dreams and your meditations, should strengthen your intuitive senses and help awaken your Self knowledge over time.

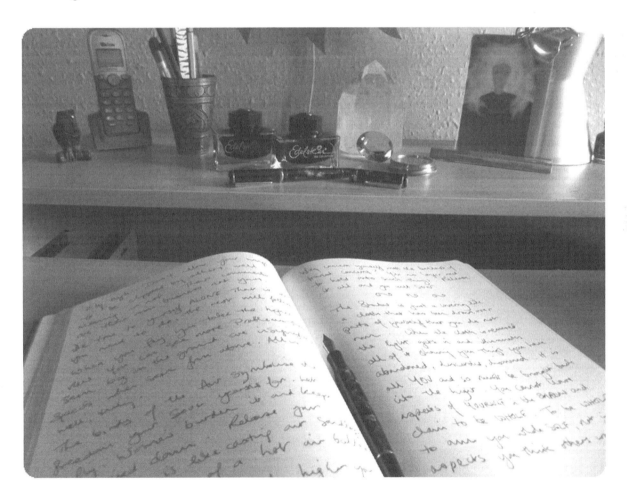

Grounding

Grounding is the foundation of a healthy energy system and everyone can benefit from it. All healers must be very aware of their grounded state, as to heal effectively, safely and in a sustainable way requires the flow of healing energy through a well-grounded energy system.

By grounding I am referring to the connection of your energy field to that of the Earth. This connection allows you to draw from the abundant source of Mother Earth's energy whilst at the same time ensuring that you do not accumulate excess energy. You can think of this like the earth wire for electricity, excess energy is safely dissipated into the ground so you are not overloaded. Being well grounded helps you deal with life in a secure and rational manner.

Many people go through their lives being ungrounded. If you know people who seem to be off in a dream world, or 'dizzy', chances are their grounding is poor. Similarly people who have a tendency to be nervy, fly off the handle or get things out of proportion. Outbursts of anger are a less pleasant way that the body can discharge built up energy. Lack of grounding is also a feature of many conditions that leave people weak and listless.

You can become aware of your grounded state. Often the Earth connection takes the form of a slight buzzing, warmth, or tingling under the sole of each foot. You may also feel more stable and firm on your feet. It is useful to train yourself in this awareness. When you have practiced regularly you should find that you can ground yourself simply by thinking of grounding, or by turning your attention to the soles of your feet. This is the work of seconds, but can make a huge difference to your life.

Some methods of grounding are passive. The person being grounded doesn't consciously have to do anything. Some activities are naturally very grounding. Keen gardeners usually have a good Earth connection. Walking around barefoot is helpful, especially outdoors. Other passive methods include having something to eat or drink, or doing some exercise.

Crystals can be used in this way and it is very important as a crystal healer that you remember to ground anyone you work on. I find I need to ground most clients during their treatments and I always check they are well grounded before they leave. Strong grounding can help to 'fix' the adjustments made in the energy field during a treatment.

For people that need to reinforce their grounding on a daily basis I recommend that grounding stones are placed between the feet whilst sitting watching TV or working, however they can also be carried in pouches or worn as jewellery.

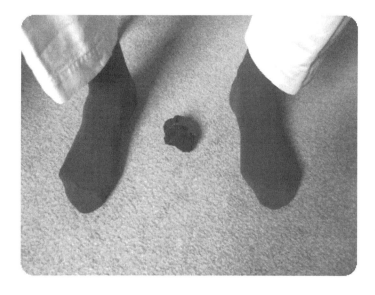

Grounding with Crystals

The best grounding stones are generally dark or earthy in colour. There are a range of placements for grounding effectively whilst lying down. You can place them under each foot, between the ankles, centrally about twelve inches below the feet or between the thighs. If you are using a crystal with a termination, such as a smoky quartz, then direct the point downwards away from the body.

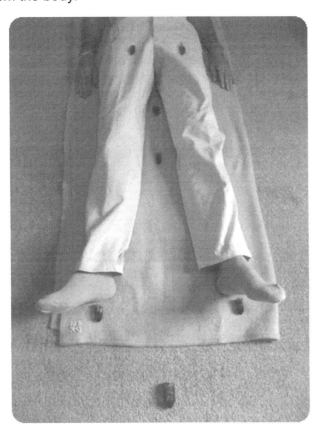

Most people only need one or two grounding stones, but some people have serious issues with their grounding and may need more to really anchor them firmly. My personal preference is to ground clients at the Earth Star which is about 12 inches between and below the feet. If your client is on a treatment couch you'd place the stone on the floor.

A strong Base chakra is important for grounding and a pair of stones placed at the tops of the thighs will support this. Although between the tops of the thighs is a good place to stimulate grounding this is a sensitive and personal part of the body, so it is wise to let the client place a crystal here and let them recover it for themselves at the end of the treatment.

If your client feels a bit 'out of it' at the end of the session you can sit them up and they can hold a grounding stone whilst they are having a glass of water and discussing their treatment. You can also place a grounding stone between their feet whilst they are sitting. This is a simple self help placement for clients who are generally ungrounded and is useful if you treat anyone who cannot lie down.

Touchstones

Hematite: a heavy metallic stone which brings you 'back down to Earth' with ease.
Smoky quartz: the most grounding member of the quartz family.
Tiger's eye: encourages a well grounded and practical approach to life.
Black tourmaline (schorl): grounding, protecting and purifying.

Grounding with Tree Energies

Trees are excellent helpers as they have their roots in the earth and their branches in the sky. In the same way we wish to connect to Spirit without losing our Earth connection.

If you are feeling 'spacey' you can imagine standing inside a hollow tree like this one and letting it help you to ground, or visualise leaning against a favourite tree. If possible go outside and lean up against a real tree, feeling its support. Even people who have great difficulties with their grounding report feeling more grounded when they connect with a tree.

A basic grounding visualisation can be helpful. Use the image of roots growing out from the sole of each foot deep down into Mother Earth and imagine them securing you firmly like a tree. When you feel your 'roots' are secure you may also visualise reaching up to the heavens as tree branches do and so you receive support from both Heaven and Earth.

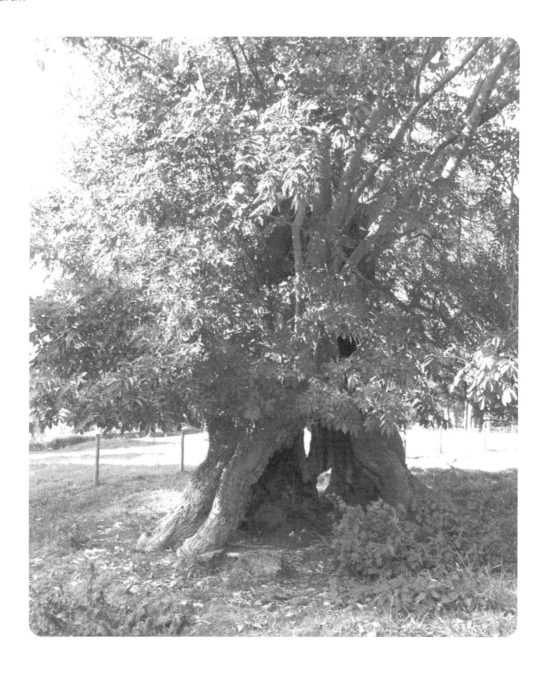

Coming to Your Centre

Having your energies centred will create a feeling of more stability, peace and harmony for yourself. By coming to centre I mean a focusing of your energy at a central point in the body. By doing this we avoid our focus being scattered and we can respond with a more coherent and balanced approach to life. You become less likely to be upset by other people and events and you can regain your equilibrium more quickly and easily when this does happen.

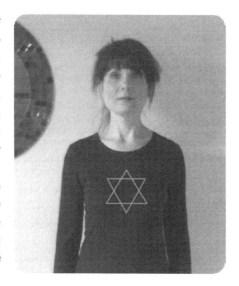

As a therapy teacher I encourage my students to centre themselves at the heart chakra as this is the balance point of the chakra system. The symbol of the heart chakra is the Seal of Solomon, which combines a triangle pointing up to the Heavens and a triangle pointing down to the Earth.

So how do you come to centre? There are several ways of achieving this state quickly and easily. You can use them daily, or as often as you need to.

Tapping

If you tap firmly (not too hard!) in the centre of your chest just below where your collarbone meets your breastbone with the fingers of one hand you will centre yourself. As a bonus you'll also stimulate the thymus gland which then helps to boost your immune system. You can either tap in one spot or tap around this area in a small circle. In healing this is referred to as 'tapping in' and is a very quick way for the therapist to check that their own energies are centred prior to a treatment.

Sound

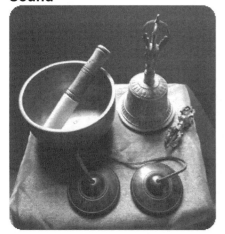

You can use a sound to bring your mind fully into the present moment. Focus on the point in the centre of your chest that is level with your physical heart. My favourite instrument for doing this are tingshas, those little cymbals sold in pairs. They are sounded by striking one gently on the rim of the other. Take a couple of slow deep breaths and then strike them just in front of your heart centre and listen until the note fades away and becomes inaudible. This is also a pleasant way to settle your energies before a meditation and to bring yourself back to normal waking consciousness following meditation.

Alternatively you could use a singing bowl, bell, or a chime. You want to find an instrument that carries a pleasant and reverberating note when played, giving a feeling of spaciousness and plenty of time to come to centre.

You can use your own voice. Toning is a very effective way to bring your focus to your centre. The bija mantra for the heart centre is 'Yam'. Either tone 'Yam' (sounds like *yahm*) as a long sound or repeat 'Yam, Yam Yam' several times until you feel your energies are centred. Think of your voice as being bell-like in its tone. Some people prefer to chant 'Om' or tone 'Ooo' or a relaxing 'Aah', try these sounds out and see what suits you.

Crystals

      Choose a cleansed quartz point with a ground base that allows it to stand upright. Sit down and place it on a table in front of you. Gaze into the quartz intending that you are connecting with its energy at your heart whilst you breathe your awareness into this chakra. The size of the crystal isn't too important it just needs to feel right for you. If you don't have a quartz point with a flat base you can stand a crystal upright in a bowl of sand. You should find you become centred within a few minutes. Alternatively simply hold a crystal at your heart centre and focus your attention on it.

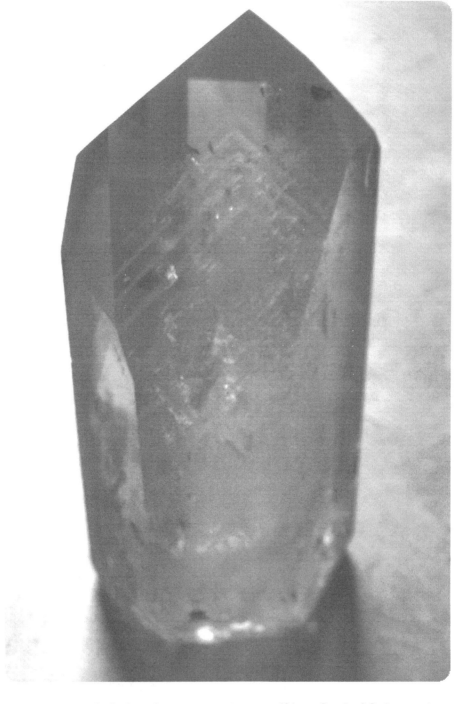

If you feel really discombobulated you can put yourself in a Seal of Solomon layout for 10-15 minutes. See the Basic Techniques section.

Shielding and Protecting your Energy

When you move unpleasant energies from a client in a healing you don't want to take them into your own system. Keep your own energy shielded and the debris will not attach to you. Anyone who works a lot with people, particularly with the sick or vulnerable, would be advised to build basic energetic protection into their routine.

Using Crystals

Many crystals have protective qualities. You can wear them as jewellery or carry them, or if you feel unsafe at night pop them under your pillow, or by the bed.

A Crystalline Shell

Visualise yourself enclosed within a crystalline shell. You can imagine these crystals as natural points, like an amethyst geode completely surrounding you, or as a layer of thousands of brightly shining faceted gemstones, such as diamonds or rubies, or as a sphere of shiny stone, like black obsidian.

You may change your crystalline protection to suit the energy of the day ahead, see what is suggested in your mind's eye. You may then choose to carry a crystal of the type you have visualised to strengthen and maintain this shield as you move through your day.

Touchstones

Black tourmaline: very strong protection, creates an 'energetic fortress' around you.
Black obsidian: imagine a shiny smooth reflective shield sealing the aura.
Labradorite: a magical colour changing stone that creates a force field around you.
Diamond: imagine thousands of faceted diamonds creating a dazzling shield.
Pyrite: visualise wearing a shiny suit of golden armour made of pyrites.

Sacred Symbols of Protection

Humankind has used symbols of protection, or amulets, for millennia. Some of the symbols in common use today date back thousands of years, such as the Ankh, the Cross, the Star of David and the Pentagram. If you believe in a symbol it is much more powerful for you personally, so it is important that you choose a protective symbol that resonates. There isn't much point wearing a Christian Cross if you have mixed feelings about Christianity, or a Pentagram if you hold 'Hammer House of Horror' views about witchcraft for example!

Detaching Your Energy

We naturally make energy connections with other people we are close to. This can happen with people you work with, family members and friends. Some will be harmonious and very light, others may be quite draining. You know how you feel when you are around certain people!

When you are working with a client energy connections may form between you. If the connections are left in place they can be draining for the therapist, particularly if the client is ill or feels needy. It is good auric hygiene to consciously release any connections at the end of a healing session.

Get into the habit of detaching energetically from your clients after they leave you. Make this part of a simple routine such as washing your hands, which is good physical and energetic hygiene, or using an essence spray, or sweeping around your aura with a blade of kyanite with the intent that you are releasing any connections you have made with the client. I disconnect from my clients as I wave them off at the door.

Putting it all Together: The Ground and Protect Visualisation

The following visualisation is excellent for maintaining a safe, grounded, centred and connected state and is good preparation for healing, but it can also be used on a daily basis and is most effective as a part of your morning routine, just like brushing your teeth. If you'd like to listen I've recorded it and put it on my YouTube channel: Lauren D'Silva

Sit comfortably with your feet flat on the floor and your back upright. You may prefer to stand up straight. Close your eyes and take a few deep breaths. Breathe in through your nose and out through your mouth. With every breath you feel more relaxed and more relaxed.

Become aware of the connection your feet are making with the floor. Take your attention to the soles of your feet.

Imagine that from the centre of each foot you can see roots growing down, like tree roots. As you watch you'll see the roots are growing longer and stronger, delving down into the ground. Continue to push your roots down deeper and deeper, longer and stronger, down into Mother Earth, until you sense you have reached the centre of the Earth, where there is an endless supply of Earth energy.

Your roots make contact with Mother Earth's energy and as they do her energy begins to flow up your roots, rising all the way up. Allow her energy to rise up through your roots, nourishing you, rising all the way up, until it makes contact with the soles of your feet.

Now allow Earth's energy to flow up through your feet, up through your lower legs, your thighs, up through your abdomen until it reaches the level of your heart centre.

Visualise Mother Earth's energy swirling in a ball in the centre of your chest and enjoy the loving warmth of her energy at your heart.

Now take your attention high above your head, where you will become aware of a bright white star. Take a strand of the white starlight and draw it down towards you. It enters through the crown of your head and fills your head, your neck, flowing downwards until it meets the Earth energy at your heart centre.

You watch as the white starlight merges and mingles with the Earth energy. Watch the pattern as they swirl together.

As the energies combine they expand and grow. They expand outwards from your heart covering the whole of your chest, and then continue to grow encompassing your whole body, and expand further still until they fill your whole aura, shaped like a great egg all around you, above your head and below your feet. Wait until your aura is filled with this bright energy.

Now get a sense of the outer edge of your aura. You are going to visualise some protection. You might picture a crystalline shell perhaps made of amethyst, diamonds, labradorite, or obsidian. You might see a long hooded cloak around you, or a golden membrane. You may find that your protection changes from day to day. Your Higher Self knows what you need to keep your energies safe. Form a clear picture of this protection surrounding your entire aura. Know that it will allow positive energy to come through to you, but will repel any unhelpful energies. When you have that clear picture know that your protection will remain in place for the rest of the day.

Now let the images fade and take your attention back to your breathing, in through your nose and out through your mouth. Become aware of the chair supporting you and the floor beneath your feet. Become more aware of the room around you and any sounds from outside. Open your eyes and give yourself a stretch before you continue with your day.

Keeping Your Energies Fresh and Clean

Sometimes we are so immersed in difficult or challenging situations that we feel energetically off colour when we get home, as though some of that unwholesome energy has rubbed off onto us. At other times we are processing our own old hurts and unhelpful emotions and need help to release the energy out of our system. Just as we keep our physical bodies cleansed of sweat and grime, so we can benefit from an energetic cleanse. There are lots of tried and tested methods of cleansing. Experiment and use the ones that feel helpful to you.

If you feel you are picking up a lot of heavy energy on a regular basis take a good look at your diet, thought patterns, lifestyle and way of working. It is likely that something needs to change and your aura needs to be strengthened. You may ask for professional help and book some sessions with an experienced healer if you feel you need more support. My husband Steve Deeks-D'Silva is a Shaman specialising in the distant removal of stubborn, difficult energies and his contact details are available at the end of the manual should you ever need them.

Using Water

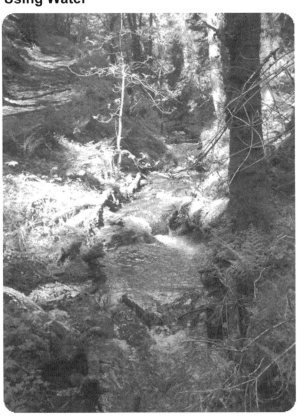

Keeping physically clean is closely allied to keeping energetically clean and a shower or bath is a good first step if you are feeling energetically heavy. I always take a shower and wash my hair in the morning on days when I am teaching or healing so that I am physically clean from top to toe.

If you shower visualise the water flowing through your energy field carrying away any negativity down the plughole with it. You may imagine that the water is coloured if you wish to add an extra dimension to the experience. Violet or electric blue are very cleansing colours.

If you prefer a bath you may like to try crystal bathing and place a few resilient tumblestones in the bath with you. For deep cleansing add a handful of sea or rock salt to the water and dissolve it well. Salt has long been renowned for its cleansing properties. Epsom salts are also known for their detoxification properties. Avoid running the bath too hot as you may feel a bit light-headed after a cleansing bath. It is best to give yourself time to settle and relax afterwards. For this reason I prefer to take a cleansing bath in the evening.

A quick cleanse that can provide instant relief and doesn't look too strange even in a public washroom is to hold your wrists under cool running water. Imagine you are being thoroughly cleansed as all the blood in your body is circulated past your wrists.

If you aren't close to running water you can visualise paddling in a stream, standing under a waterfall, or swimming in the ocean.

Touchstones

Amethyst: is cleansing, aids peaceful relaxation and quiets your mind as you bathe.
Rose Quartz: makes a bath into a time of self care and boosts self worth.
Aventurine: helps you to relax and come back to centre as you soak.

Get Outside into Nature

Some places are particularly cleansing and recharging. A walk by the sea invigorates mind, body and spirit. Alternatively any other stretch of clean running water is cleansing and waterfall energy can be wonderfully refreshing. Hilltops are usually healthy places to go as there is more chance of a breeze which can 'blow away the cobwebs'. Woodlands usually have an uplifting energy. Even in a City it is good to get away from the streets and into a park, or just to sit out in the garden.

If you cannot get outside you can visualise walking through beautiful sunlit woods or along the seashore. Imagine the breeze blowing around you carrying any heaviness away. Visualise breathing in the fresh air and imagine the sunshine dissolving any cloudy energy from your aura.

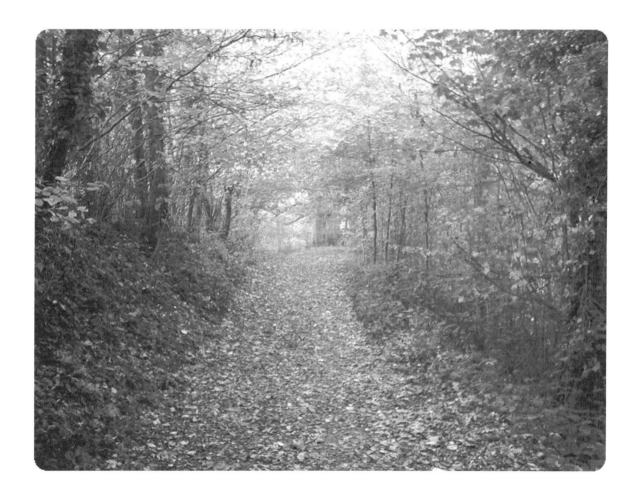

Breathing

Most of us are in the bad habit of shallow breathing. We don't inflate or deflate our lungs fully. The result is that we don't use the available prana, chi, or life force energy that is in abundance all around us.

Rapid shallow breathing is an agitated form of breathing designed to keep your mind and body on alert. Like other physical manifestations of stress it puts us in survival mode which is essential when faced with a real threat, but keeping our body on alert when the only 'threat' is a deadline or a meeting is not healthy. If you are feeling anxious or agitated then deeper breathing, even for a few minutes will help to calm you. Just encouraging someone to breathe more deeply and slowly can bring them out of a panic attack.

It is useful to breathe deeply and slowly when healing. This increases our intake of life force energy and encourages the client to relax and breathe more deeply too.

Our brains are affected by our breathing patterns. Brainwaves are measured in Hz. There are four main brainwave patterns:

Delta state is characterised by deep meditation and deep sleep: 0.5Hz - 4Hz. Delta waves give us a 'vacation' and deep peace. It is a healing and regeneration frequency. I've found that when clients relax this deeply they tend to have profound healing experiences. Allow extra time for coming back to normal waking consciousness at the end of the session.

Theta state is found in sleep and meditation: 4Hz - 7Hz. It is characteristic of the surfacing/going under phase of sleep. It enhances intuition and psychic perception. This state is often accessed during a crystal healing and clients may report seeing coloured light and images.

Alpha state is dreaming and relaxation: 7Hz - 12 Hz. Most clients will easily relax into this state during a treatment.

Beta state is our normal waking awareness, the higher the Hz the more alert and focussed: 13Hz-40HZ. Where clients are determined to stay alert they can block their own healing. Encourage 'watchful' clients to close their eyes and take a few deep breaths.

Selenite Breathing

- Hold a selenite crystal in front of your face.
- Imagine you can see the selenite enriched air sparkling with white light as you inhale it through your nostrils.
- Picture the infused air making its way into your lungs, filling them with clean sparkling energy.
- Observe the short pause which follows the in breath and drop your hands holding the selenite to your lap.
- Now visualise the air tinged with the impurities you have flushed out as it leaves your lungs and you breathe it out through your mouth.
- Observe the pause which follows and raise the selenite in front of your face before you breathe in again.
- Continue to do as many rounds of selenite breathing as feels good to you. 10 is a good number to start with.
- Check you are well grounded before you go on with your day.

Touchstones

Selenite: the cleansing, clarifying energy of selenite makes it an ally for breath work.

Incense, Smudge and Sound
These cleansing methods are discussed fully in the **Space Clearing** section at the end of the manual.

Visualisation
Your imagination can have a powerful effect on your energy. There are many different ways you can imagine being cleansed; here is a visualisation utilising crystals:

Violet Flame Visualisation with Amethyst
You will need: one amethyst point, or an amethyst cluster.

- Sit quietly with your back upright holding the amethyst in your lap with any points facing upwards. Close your eyes and take a few deep breaths.
- In your mind's eye the amethyst takes on the appearance of a violet flame. At first the flame is the same size as the amethyst, but as you watch it grows to encompass your whole body and your aura.
- Sit quietly in the violet flame and give it permission to burn away and transmute any heaviness you are holding anywhere in your energy. Imagine tongues of violet flame reaching into each of your chakras and clearing them. Feel it going into any area of your body that holds tension or pain. Release any toxic thoughts and negative emotions for transmutation in the violet flame.
- When you feel cleansed, or feel you have released enough for one session then you watch the flames withdraw back into the amethyst you are holding. Imagine you are placing a violet cloak around your head and shoulders to protect yourself.
- Take a deep breath, stretch, open your eyes. Drink a glass of water and hold a grounding stone if you feel lightheaded.

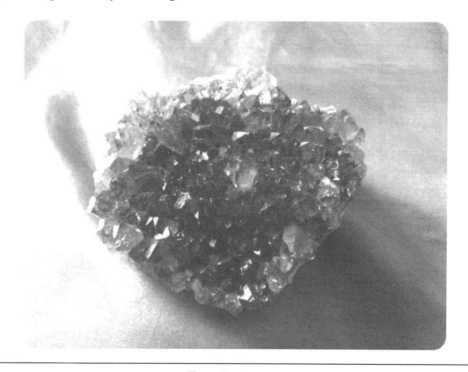

Touchstones
Amethyst: the energy of amethyst is aligned with the violet flame. If you find visualisation difficult simply hold amethyst and intend the violet flame will cleanse you.

Maintaining a Strong Energy Field

At its most basic energetic protection is about staying fit and healthy. People with a robust constitution are much less likely to pick up unpleasant energies. If your aura is strong and resilient then unpleasant energy should just bounce off you. All the usual health advice applies: regular exercise, a healthy diet, enough rest and relaxation, avoiding illegal drugs and alcohol. Never do any healing work if you have taken illegal drugs or had an alcoholic drink, make sure such substances are fully out of your system.

Be Positive

My observation is that optimists are generally healthier than pessimists. I believe that negative thinkers can't repel challenges to their systems as effectively, whether that's from a cold bug or an unhelpful energy.

Get Outside

Natural energies can really perk up your aura. When you are indoors you don't get the benefit of the full spectrum of light, so if the sun shines take the opportunity to sit or stand in it for a while and feel the rays topping your batteries up!

Stay Grounded

Practice a grounding visualisation every morning and whenever you feel at all 'spacey'. Eventually you should be able to just think 'grounding' and feel yourself connect to the Earth. Carry hematite or another grounding stone with you if you have difficulty with your visualisation. **If you skipped the previous section on grounding go back and read it now!**

Avoid EMFs and Geopathic Stress

Your aura will be stronger if you limit the time you spend in close proximity to electromagnetic fields (EMFs) such as those generated by computers. Don't carry your mobile phone in your pocket and don't leave electrical equipment switched on near your bed, not even on 'standby'. EMFs can weaken your energy field. Avoid sleeping or sitting for long periods in Geopathic Stress (GS). There is more information on both of these topics in the chapter on the Energy of the Space.

Energetic Support

If we are honest most of us are not on top form and in peak health every day. It isn't practical to withdraw from the world every time you feel less than 100%, so it is useful to create a team of energetic supporters that bolster your natural energy when you need them. My favourite supporters are crystals and gem essences. You choose the support that feels good to you.

Many crystals have energy strengthening and protective qualities. Wear your chosen energy support crystal as jewellery, or carry the crystal/s in a pouch or in your pocket.

There are many ranges of readymade essences available either to take as drops or to mist through your aura. I particularly like Alaskan Essences 'Soul Support' spray and I also make my own gem essences and dowse which I need. Gem essence making is taught in the TSCT Diploma course.

Touchstones

Carnelian: an encouraging energy, giving a feeling of 'I can do that!'
Red jasper: fortifying, strengthening energy.
Iron pyrites: dynamic, sparkling, confidence boosting energy.

Chapter Three:
Care for your Crystals

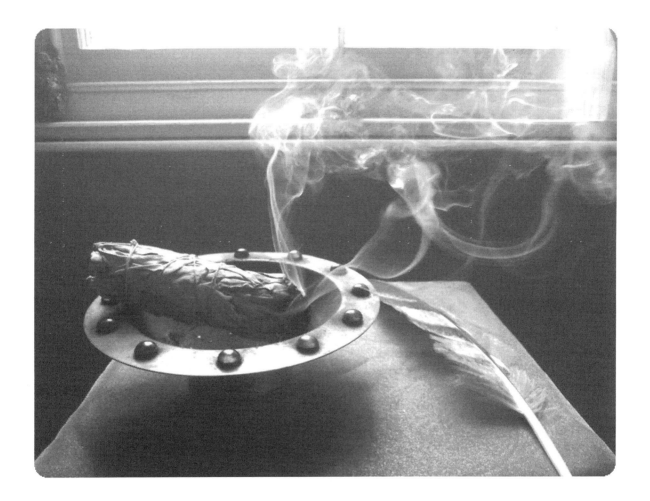

Cleansing Crystals

Why bother? Crystals each have their own energy field. Just as with people the energy field of a crystal can absorb other energies. We use this feature as crystal healers to work with the stones and build up positive healing vibrations; however the crystal is also susceptible to less helpful vibrations. It may have lifted some heavy energy away from someone, or picked up electromagnetic radiation from televisions, computers, mobile phones and other electronic devices.

When we utilise crystals for healing we are using them to bring about change in our client's energy field. If the crystal is holding onto unhelpful energies then the result may be far from therapeutic!

When should I Cleanse my Crystals?

When you purchase them:

Most crystals are mined, many in third world countries. Sadly the people doing the mining may not be working in conditions conducive to the most loving 'birth'. Crystals may be handled roughly and most have a long journey to make. They may then have waited in a warehouse before being bought by the retailer and then may have sat on a shop shelf and been handled by dozens of people before you purchased them.

Although some reputable sellers know about cleansing and cleanse all of their stock on a regular basis, you cannot know who has touched them and the vibrations they carry; therefore it is always advisable to cleanse your crystals after purchase.

When you use them for healing:

When you have been using crystals in a healing you may have loosened some heavy energy from your client. If you don't cleanse your crystals following the healing you may transfer this onto your next client. Therefore you should always cleanse crystals following a healing.

When you use them around the home:

Crystals which have been sitting by electrical equipment will need regular cleansing, as will other crystals which have been strategically placed to absorb unhelpful vibrations. Crystals will also pick up on the atmosphere in a room. Cleanse your crystals and the room thoroughly after any argument, illness or after difficult visitors. You may want to institute a regular cleanse of all of your 'ornamental' crystals, perhaps using the first of the month as your reminder.

When you wear them or carry them:

Wearing crystal jewellery is an effective and attractive way of bringing crystal energies into your daily life, however if you neglect to cleanse your jewellery the crystals can become overloaded. In normal use a weekly cleansing is enough, however if you are poorly, going through a patch of upset or turmoil, or using the jewellery to protect you from difficult energies then you would be wiser to give them a daily cleanse.

Methods of Cleansing Your Crystals

Running Water:

Hold the crystal under running water. If you have several stones to cleanse you can use the little net bags you get with laundry tablets, this will also prevent them escaping! I've used the inner plastic colander from a salad spinner for years. It isn't pretty, but it is practical. Tap water will do the job, but a clean stream, spring, or waterfall is lovely and will fill the crystals with the energy of living waters too. You must make sure that the crystals are not going to be damaged by water. Selenite, sulphur and halite are common examples of water sensitive crystals.

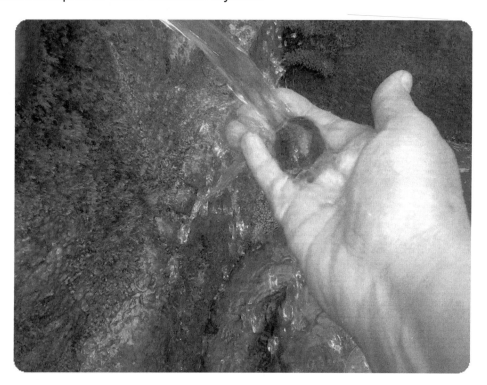

Using Soapy Water

Where crystals are physically grimy use of soapy water is appropriate. I use a mild detergent and warm water to wash the stones and I then rinse them in clean warm water and lay them to dry in the sun, or use a towel. Do not do this with any water sensitive crystals.

Gem Essences

Spraying a fine mist of an essence created with cleansing in mind will cleanse crystals very quickly. This is particularly useful for cleansing crystals between clients, where you need to use the same crystals again and haven't time for the other methods. You can also run a small bowl of water and add a few drops of a cleansing essence to give your crystals a good soak. Be sure only to use this method for crystals that are not damaged by water.

Intention

When other methods of cleansing are not convenient you can use the focused power of your intention to cleanse crystals. Hold the crystal in your hands, look at it and visualise it being cleansed by a stream of white light.

Cleansing with Smoke

Follow the detailed directions in the section on Space Clearing. You can waft smudge over the crystals using a feather. You can either let incense fill the whole room or 'wash' the crystals by holding them in the smoke. I use a basket so that I can cleanse several crystals at once. This is my preferred method at the end of the day after I have been seeing clients. Both my healing room and the crystals are cleansed ready for the next day.

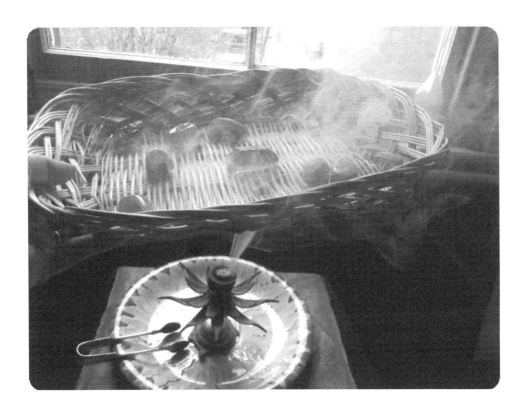

Heavy Duty Cleansing

It is appropriate to use these deeper cleansing methods if you notice a crystal has a very 'heavy' or 'sticky' energy about it that does not clear despite using several of the methods already described.

Cleansing with Salt

Salt is a traditional cleansing agent. It has strong absorbent properties both physically and on an energetic level. Place crystals in a bowl of sea salt. Use your intuition or dowsing to guide you to the length of time to leave them. Be aware that salt can damage some crystals. Do not use this method on opals for example, as salt will absorb the water content, which makes them iridescent. You need to throw the salt away after use.

Burying in Earth

Crystals come from the ground and have grown within the natural energies of the planet. This method is a useful deep cleansing solution to be used where a stone has been traumatised and feels very unhealthy. You may even decide to release it back into the care of Mother Earth and let it go. Bury the stone and label the spot well if you want to be able to retrieve it. Leave it to rest. It may need days, weeks, or maybe even months to recuperate. You can always check on its progress, give it a wash and rebury it if necessary.

Charging Crystals

Some crystals, once cleansed feel 'raring to go'. Others still feel like they need something else. Charging crystals fills their structure with Universal energy and most crystals can benefit from being charged when you first buy them and then at intervals whenever their energy feels a little dulled or tired.

Different crystals prefer different methods of charging. You will need to use your intuition to decide what is best.

Charging with Sunlight

Most crystals enjoy a good sunbathe. Pick a bright sunny day and put them out in the sunshine. You might only need to leave them out for an hour or two, or you might need to leave them all day. Intuition and dowsing are your best guides. If you live somewhere without a garden, or if your crystals might 'walk' if you left them outside, then you can use a sunny windowsill, but be aware that the light is filtered by the glass so this isn't quite as effective. Amethyst, fluorite and a few other stones will fade if left in sunlight over a long period of time.

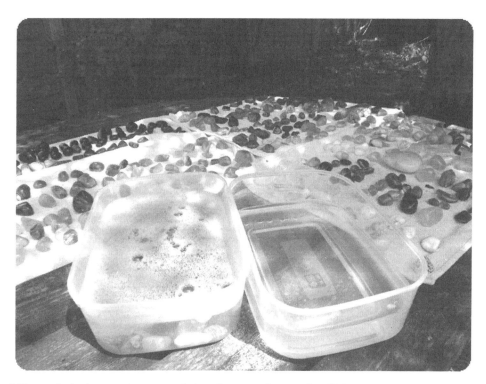

Although I cleanse my crystals after each use I still have a big crystal washing and charging session at least once or twice a year to get rid of any physical dirt and give my whole collection an energy boost. I carry everything out into the garden. I have a couple of bowls of lukewarm water, one with a mild detergent and one plain for rinsing and I carefully wash all but the water sensitive crystals, then spread them out in the sunshine on my garden table to sunbathe. It takes some hours, but it is well worth it.

Charging with Moonlight

Crystals with quieter yin or female energies may prefer to moonbathe. Pick a clear night ideally when the moon is waxing or full. Again an hour or two may be enough, but you are quite likely to need to leave them out all night as the moon's energy is more subtle. Receptive crystals such as crystal balls and selenite or moonstone enjoy this method, but check the weather forecast for selenite as it is water sensitive, a moonlit windowsill is a safer option.

Charging with Crystals

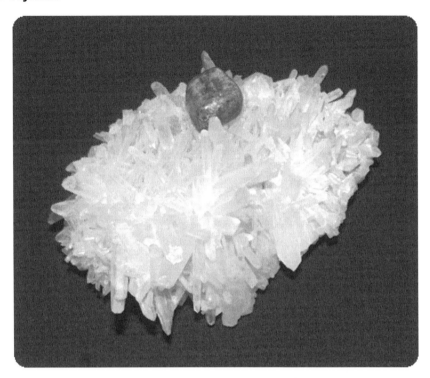

A quartz crystal cluster or amethyst bed can be used for charging. My husband Steve designed copper and crystal charging plates especially for this purpose; they are also excellent for sending absent healing. You can get a similar effect by placing six cleansed and charged quartz points evenly around the chosen crystal, points inwards. Remember the charging crystals will also need periodic cleansing and charging!

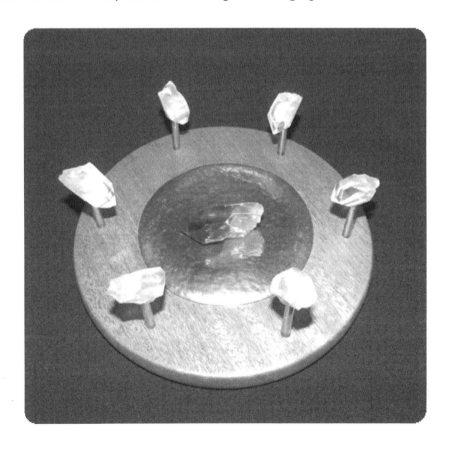

Chapter Four:
Choosing Crystals

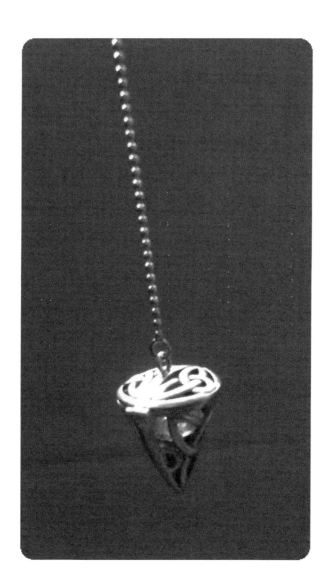

Choosing Your Crystals

Choosing a crystal for healing is an intuitive process; even when you have learned about crystal attributes the best crystal for the job may not be the one that your logical mind suggests.

Before you start choosing you need to make sure you have grounded, connected to your Higher Self and centred yourself. If you skip this basic preparation you are less likely to make good choices. Now consider what you would like to use the crystal for. Is it a crystal for the day ahead, or is it to meditate with, to place on an ache, or for a specific issue a client has presented with?

As a therapist you need to ensure that your intention is clear and aligned to the highest good for all concerned in any given situation. This will help you make wise choices.

Selecting Crystals by Hand Scanning

Sensing crystals with your hands will increase your awareness of subtle energies. These instructions give you a good chance of sensing some crystal energies on your first attempt, but don't worry if it takes you longer. With experience you'll probably become more aware and more able to differentiate between these subtle sensations.

- Wash and dry your hands if possible, or give your hands a shake to remove any sticky energies.
- Remember to ground, connect, centre and protect your energy field.
- Rub your hands together briskly. This activates the minor chakras in the palms of the hands. You may notice they tingle.
- Focus your intention upon finding the most helpful crystal for your chosen purpose.
- Pass your left hand over the crystals. Most people find one hand is more receptive than the other; it is often the left hand as that is connected to the more creative side of your brain. Try with your right hand too and see if you notice any difference between them.
- Pay attention to any subtle changes. People sense crystal energies in different ways. You may notice sensations such as a magnetic pull, a change in vibration, a temperature change, or a breeze.
- Choose the crystal that feels like it is attracting your attention the most. If your hand is drawn to several crystals you may want to spread them out and scan them again to find the best one to use.

Intuition

As you become used to working with crystals you will probably find that you are confident enough to be guided by your intuition and will just 'know' which stone you need. You may get an image of the stone in your mind's eye, or its name might pop into your mind. You can also make good choices by gazing at your crystals. Steve wears glasses and to select crystals he removes them. He finds the right crystal will light up for him and have a glow around it.

- Remember to ground, connect, centre and protect before you start.
- Set your intention.
- Gaze gently across your crystals
- Notice a crystal that stands out amongst the rest

Pendulum Dowsing

Pendulum dowsing is a useful skill and just about anyone can learn it. Basic dowsing gives a yes/no response to questions asked. As a crystal therapist a pendulum will be a key part of your toolkit. Just about any small weighted object on the end of a string or chain can act as a pendulum. When crystal healing I use a crystal pendulum, but to give a yes/no response any pendulum will do. Caught without a pendulum at a workshop one time I threaded a seashell on a piece of cotton; it actually made a beautiful pendulum and several people asked me where I got it!

Your choice of crystal pendulum is personal. I like to use clear quartz as it is so versatile and I prefer simple single stone pendulums rather than the fancy multi-stone ones on the market.

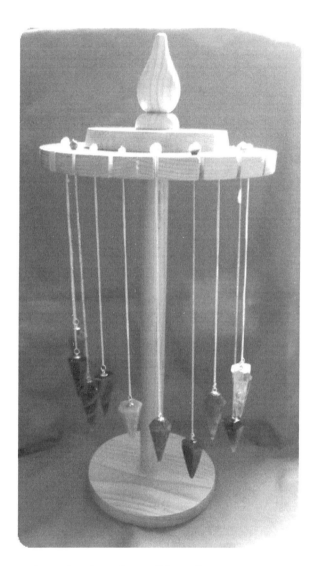

You can dowse to ask almost anything; however you are likely to become less accurate when questions have too much personal importance for you. Neutrality is vital. If you ask an emotionally loaded question such as, "Does so and so love me?" your conscious mind will most likely influence the answer, possibly giving you a false positive because you are willing it to be true, or a false negative because you are doubting and insecure. Likewise dowsing lottery numbers is something lots of people have tried. Proficient dowsers would all be rich if that one worked! When you dowse you need to be operating from a Higher Self perspective. Winning the lottery for most people is not in your highest interest whatever your ego self thinks!

Here's a step by step approach to pendulum dowsing for the first time:

- First prepare your energies: ground, connect, centre and protect.
- Hold your pendulum in one hand by the chain and let it swing gently. Although you can dowse using a pendulum from a standstill it is easier at the beginning if there is already some movement. Keep your hand and arm relaxed; tensing up will prevent the pendulum swinging freely.
- Ask a question in your mind for which you know the answer is a definite 'yes'. I might ask, "Is my name Lauren?" for example. Watch how the pendulum responds. The swing will probably change.
- You will most likely feel very excited at this point; it looks so magical! Just remember that you really are moving the pendulum, it isn't being moved by a supernatural force, simply by small unconscious muscle movements in your arm. The pendulum is a way of you accessing the wisdom of your Higher Self through these small muscle movements.
- Now ask a question, for which you know the answer is false for example, 'Am I called Arthur?' and again observe the swing. It will probably change.
- Continue to ask questions for which you know the answers until you have established how the pendulum will swing to indicate a 'yes' response and how it will swing to indicate a 'no'.
- Once you have established your 'yes' and 'no' swings you can start to use your pendulum to choose crystals and to ask questions which can be answered with a simple yes or no.

Dowsing is not infallible, but in skilled hands it can be remarkably accurate.

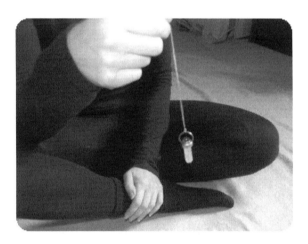

Choosing Crystals by Dowsing

Now you have established a yes and a no swing you can use the pendulum to choose crystals. Form a basic question such as, "Will this crystal help me meditate?" Now you can look at a selection of crystals in front of you and make eye contact with ones which draw your attention, whilst holding your pendulum in a neutral swing, i.e. neither your yes nor your no swing. When you make eye contact with a crystal that would be helpful your pendulum will change its swing to a yes. Some people like to combine pendulum dowsing with hand scanning and use their free hand to move across the crystals as they dowse. Others like to hold the pendulum directly over the crystals as they dowse. Try each approach and see what suits you best. As a beginner allow time for the pendulum to respond. This will get quicker with practice.

Using Dowsing Charts and Arcs

Dowsing charts are a very versatile and useful way of working with your pendulum. Dowsing charts are usually circular or semi-circular and have divisions with a different option given in each segment. They are used in various therapies, so you may see someone use a dowsing arc to work out what supplements or essences you need for example.

You can custom create a chart for almost anything which has a range of options to choose between, for example writing the crystal healing techniques you have learned onto a dowsing chart will help you to choose the most appropriate one for your client. If you don't have enough options to fill all the segments then space them evenly around the chart to make dowsing easier.

When you use dowsing charts place them on a flat surface. Ensure you have prepared yourself energetically to dowse. Hold your pendulum above the chart setting it in motion in a back forth swing. Intend that you will be shown the most appropriate option and allow the pendulum to move until its swing rests over a particular segment. At this point you can read off the option. Dowsing over charts becomes quick and efficient with practice.

One of the most versatile charts is numbered. This can be used to discern how many minutes a stone placement needs to be left for, how long to lie in a crystal net, or how many hours or days to leave distant healing set up for example.

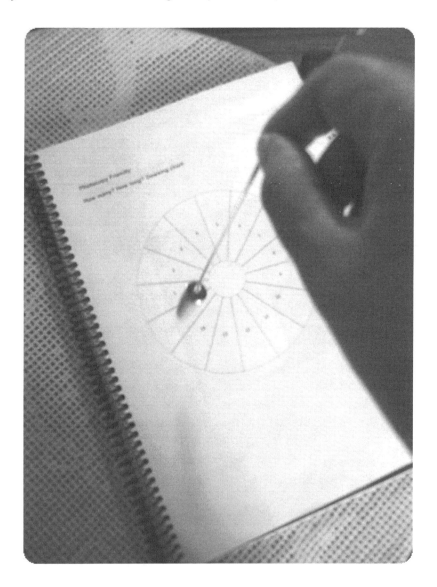

Photocopy Friendly

How many? How long? Dowsing chart

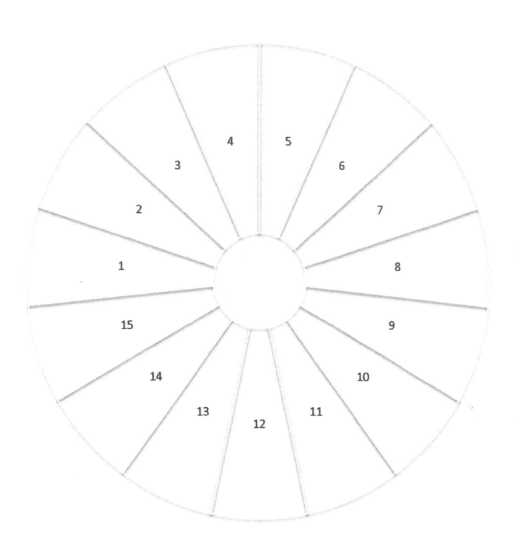

Photocopy Friendly

Blank Dowsing Chart

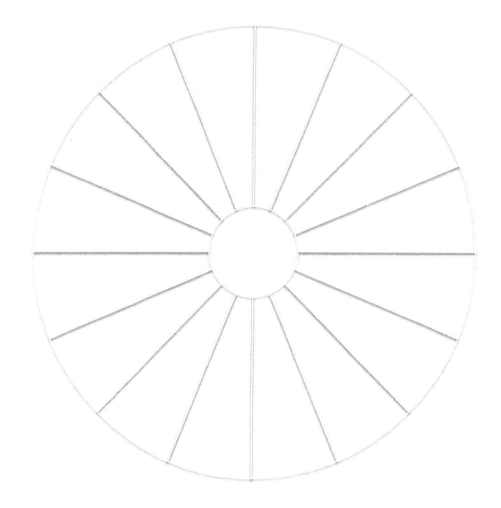

Chapter Five:
Getting to Know your Crystal Allies

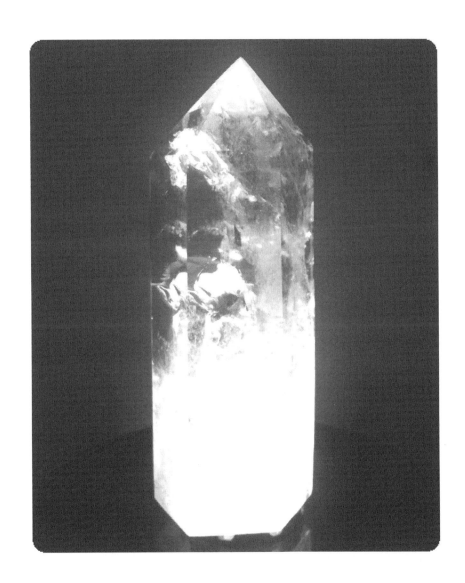

Attuning to Your Crystals

Attuning to a crystal literally means tuning into its energies. It refers to the process of getting to know a crystal, which goes beyond and is more subtle than looking it up in a reference book. Every crystal of a certain type, for example clear quartz, will share characteristics with every other crystal of that type. However every crystal has its own individual feel too. This is similar to the way all natural groupings work; all oak trees have shared and individual characteristics, all cats, or all people for that matter.

There are many ways to get to know your crystals and you will probably develop your own preferences. First ensure you have cleansed your crystal. Here are some suggestions to get you started:

- Sit quietly with the crystal in the palm of your hand and notice any sensations, images, messages or colours.
- Sit with the stone in front of you and have a piece of paper and pen to hand. Let your mind free-associate and write down any words that come to mind.
- Sit with the stone in front of you and sketch or paint it, noticing how you feel as you do this.
- Place the stone beneath your pillow and note any changes to your sleep pattern, or your dreams.
- Carry the stone around with you in your pocket, or in a pouch. Note any changes to the way you normally feel or behave.
- Use the 'Crystal Cave' visualisation.

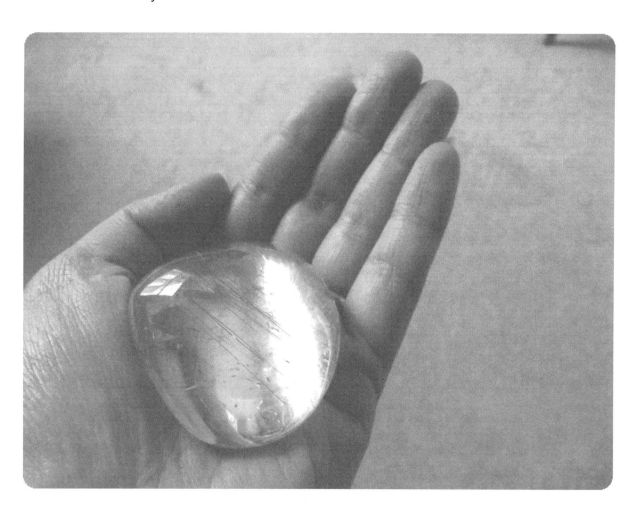

The Crystal Cave Visualisation

This visualisation will help you attune to any crystal on an intuitive level. I have recorded the visualisation if you prefer to listen to it.

Hold your chosen stone in your hands, having inspected it closely, noticing colour, shape, weight, texture, pattern and so on. Sit or lie down comfortably.

We begin in a sunny meadow. This is your 'safe haven' and you can visit it whenever you want. It takes no time at all to get there, just close your eyes, breathe and imagine it as richly as you can. Use all your senses: notice the green of the grass, the blue sky, the bright wild flowers, the colourful butterflies. Breathe in the fresh air and the delicate scent of grass, listen to the sound of the birds singing, feel the warmth of the sun and a gentle breeze on your skin. Enjoy being in this lovely place.

You can hear the sound of waves in the distance. You follow a path through the meadow which leads you to a cliff edge. Looking down you find steps cut into the cliff and you make your way down them.

At the bottom you find yourself on a beach. Notice the pebbles and the sand underfoot, the waves rolling in on the shore. In your mind's eye place the stone onto the beach. As you watch it grows, larger and larger until eventually your stone is larger than you are.

You now walk around the stone asking to be shown a way inside. The stone will show you. Sometimes it is a crevice, sometimes a doorway, a tunnel, or sometimes it simply lets you move through its walls. Continue inside until you reach the middle.

At the centre of your stone you really begin to find out about it. What are the walls like, the roof, the floor? Maybe the crystal guardian is present? Is there a message for you or an impression of what the stone would like to help you with? Is there an object in the stone? Can you examine it?

Spend time exploring or relaxing in the crystal cave.

When you are ready come out by the way you entered. First thank any guardian you met for being there. Once outside you turn to face the stone and watch as it shrinks again. Eventually it returns to its original size and you pick it back up in your hand. You return to the cliff. Make your way back up the steps and find yourself once more in the sunny meadow. When you are ready take a few deep breaths, stretch and open your eyes.

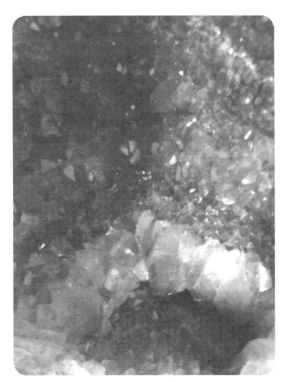

Dedicating Your Crystals

Many healers dedicate all their crystals. This is a matter of personal belief and choice. Some may dedicate their crystals to work 'in love and light' or for 'the highest good of all', others may dedicate their crystals to work with them in their devotion to a specific deity. You might want to consider forming a ritual of dedication for each new crystal as it joins your collection, or just dedicate specific crystals, such as a crystal you use on an altar.

Your dedication ritual can be as elaborate or simple as you feel is right for you and the crystal. It may just be a form of words you speak over your crystals, or you may create a more complex ceremony.

One of my former students works with the energy of Kuan Yin. She introduces all of her new crystals to a beautiful statue of Kuan Yin at her altar and they sit with the Goddess for a week or two until they feel blessed and ready to join the rest of her collection. For more information about setting up a crystal altar see the section on The Energy of Space.

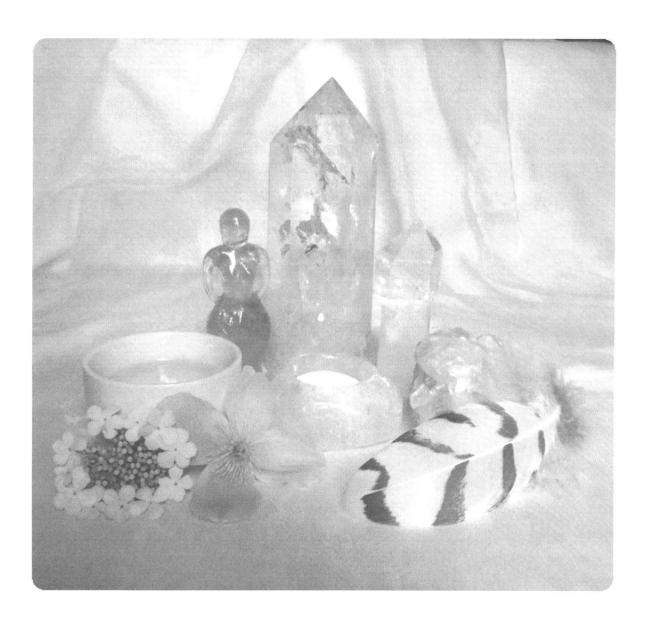

Programming Your Crystals

The basis of programming crystals lies in formulating a clear intention, then introducing it into a quartz crystal in a focused and coherent manner. Quartz crystals can hold programmes in a holographic manner. As quartz has a tendency to amplify whatever it comes into contact with it is wise to only programme crystals when you are feeling positive and when you have given a reasonable amount of thought to the programme. Your clear intention is the key to successful programming. Remember the old adage, "Be careful what you wish for."

You must decide whether it feels right for you to programme a crystal for someone else, or whether to accept one that has already been programmed. I prefer to teach others how to programme a crystal for themselves.

Your program can be formed as a picture rather than words; I like to combine words and pictures. Healing programmes can be created to treat specific health issues through the use of positive affirmations and images. By keeping the crystal upon one's person you are continually bathed in the energy of the crystal's programme. Alternatively place a programmed crystal in an appropriate part of your home, where you will see it often. Remember you will still need to cleanse programmed crystals regularly. Normal cleansing will not remove the programme.

Method of Programming

- First, determine what you would like to programme the crystal with. Get as clear as possible so that your intention is not muddied. Writing it down and checking that your programme cannot be misinterpreted by the Universe is a good idea. You may also picture the desired outcome in your mind's eye.

- If you don't believe the result you desire is possible for you then it won't be, so keep refining your intention and working on your thoughts in a positive manner until you have cleared any dominant counter-intentions out of the way.

- Choose the right crystal to take the programme. You need to find a piece of clear quartz which feels like it is in harmony with your intention. Sit with it and attune to it to check that this feels appropriate.

- Pick a time when you will not be disturbed. Place your written intention in front of you. Find the facet of the crystal that seems to be the best 'window' into the interior. Hold the crystal in front of you where you can gaze into it.

- Let your attention move into the crystal. Transfer your intended programme into your crystal using your chosen words and images. Know your desired outcome is being manifested within your crystal. When it feels like your programme has 'taken', thank the crystal and then withdraw your attention.

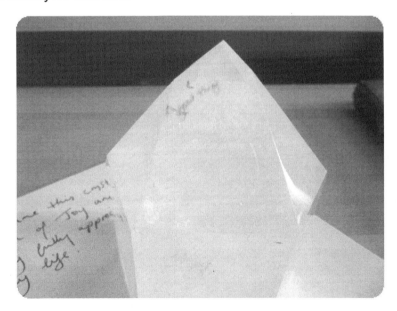

Other Types of Programming

The energies of one's favourite place in Nature, the vibrations from a particular tree, a stream, or the earthiness of a cave can all be connected with through programming a crystal:

- Choose a suitable crystal for programming.
- Go to your chosen location and respectfully ask for permission to programme your crystal with this energy. Wait for an intuitive 'yes'. If you sense a 'no' then stop at this point.
- Place the crystal in a spot that feels right to you.
- Intuit how long you need to leave the crystal in situ for.
- When the programme has 'taken' you can pick up your crystal and offer your thanks to the place.
- You may like to leave a small gift as an exchange. You might tie a coloured ribbon to a tree branch or leave a small crystal. You could gift a flower, a pinch of tobacco or cornmeal.

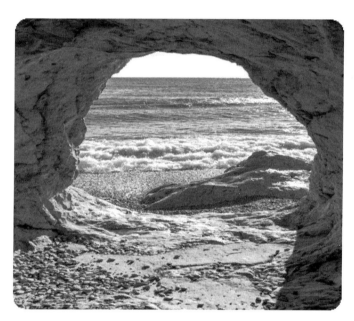

Loving bonds between people can be strengthened by exchange of crystals. As the giver, you could visualise an image of yourself looking happy and loving in the stone and acknowledge the energy you share with the recipient. The carrier of the stone will then find it easy to connect with your energy when they are away from you. This is a way for lovers to stay 'in easy energetic contact' even when they have to be apart, or for teenagers going away to live independently for the first time to maintain the energy support of a loving parent. Gemstone jewellery, gifts and in particular love tokens have been used in this way for a very long time. Trust and integrity is important here!

Erasing Programmes

Ideally you will have thought carefully about programming any crystal and will not need to erase your programme. With a well programmed crystal, normal cleansing will not remove the programme. To erase a programme you need to go through your usual programming procedure. Formulate the intent to 'erase the existing programme'. You might imagine the images fading out to white light as you do this, or any words dissolving to nothingness. This process should always be followed by cleansing and charging the crystal. Go back into the crystal and check it feels like a 'clean sheet' when you are done.

Chapter Six:
Basic Crystal Healing Techniques

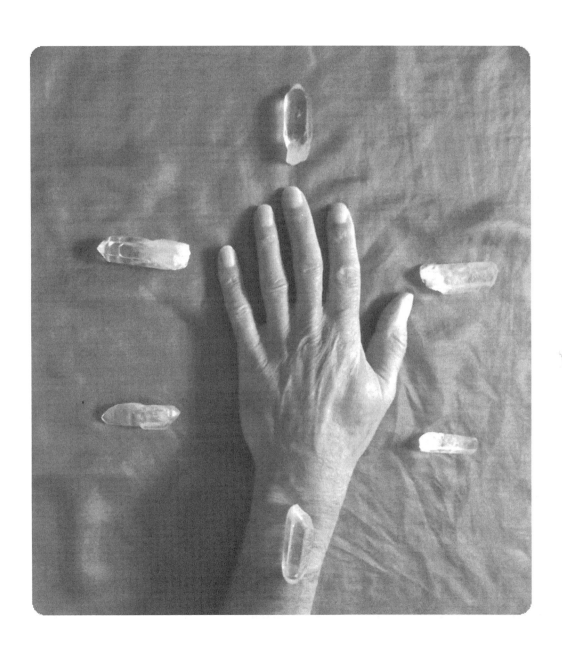

Preparing Your Client for their Healing

After an initial discussion with your client about their needs you should ask them to remove their spectacles and wristwatches if they wear them, plus take any mobile phones out of pockets and switch them off. Jewellery may also need to be removed. My clients usually keep their wedding rings and engagement rings on and if they have crystal jewellery such as a necklace I will dowse to check whether it will interfere with the treatment and ask for it to be removed if so. Some clients may wear a lot of jewellery in which case it is better to remove it. Have a place where you can put these personal items down safely. These guidelines apply to you as a healer too, aside from spectacles; it is useful to be able to see what you are doing!

If your client is made comfortable then they will relax more readily and be more receptive to the crystalline energies. If you are working on the floor use a yoga mat and blankets to provide a bit of softness. Check whether your client prefers one or two pillows. A leg roll, or bolster under the knees takes pressure off the lower back.

You may like to invest in a treatment couch as will this bring your client up to a more comfortable level for you to work. It looks professional and will save your back, also some clients may find it hard to get up and down from the floor.

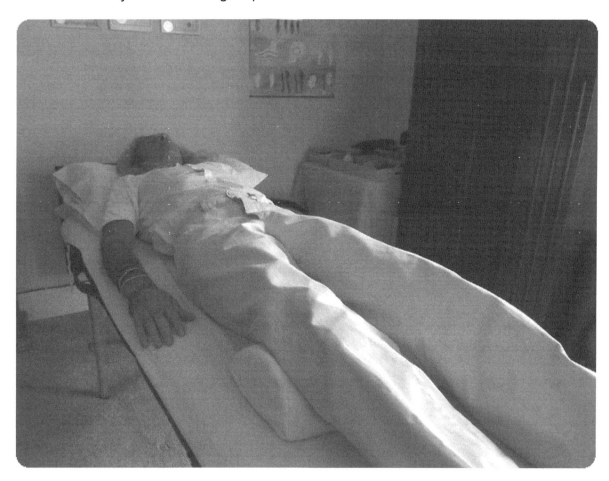

Using Quartz Points

Points direct energy and can be used to release stale energy from the body or to bring fresh energy in. They are versatile and it is worth investing in at least six to eight evenly sized quartz points.

Energy Booster: Working with Hand Held Quartz Points

One of the simplest things you can do for yourself or a client is to boost the natural flow of energy around the body using two quartz points. You can do this whilst the client is lying down for their treatment, or when sitting, and it is easy to do at home. It is especially helpful in situations where the client feels lethargic, tired and has low energy.

Hold one crystal in the left hand pointing towards the wrist and one in the right hand pointing towards the fingers. The hands can then be gently closed around the points. Points can be left in place like this throughout a treatment if it feels right and is comfortable for the client.

The left hand is the more receptive hand, hence the point bringing energy inwards, whereas the right hand is the more giving hand and so the point is directed outwards. You may notice this difference between your hands when you are working with energy.

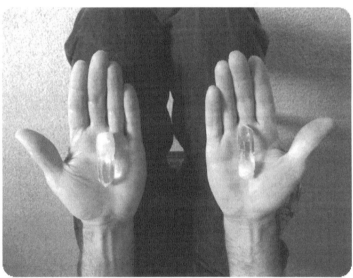

Headache Relief

Headaches can be caused by congested energy in and around the crown chakra, often created by anxious, worried or depressive thinking. Releasing some of this stagnant energy with three quartz crystals pointing outwards from the crown may bring relief.

This is also a layout to try if your thoughts are going round and round and you can't switch off from them. 5 to 10 minutes should be long enough.

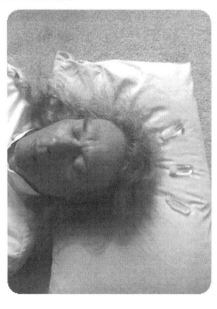

The Seal of Solomon

The 6 pointed star is an ancient and very protective sacred shape, also known as the Star of David, which symbolises the perfectly balanced energies of male and female and Heaven and Earth. When you place quartz points to face outwards they help to release old energies that are not needed and when they face inwards they recharge with fresh energy.

You will need a blanket or a yoga mat to spread on the floor and six fairly evenly sized cleansed quartz points, an inch or so long. If you are working on a couch you can place the crystals around the couch on the floor.

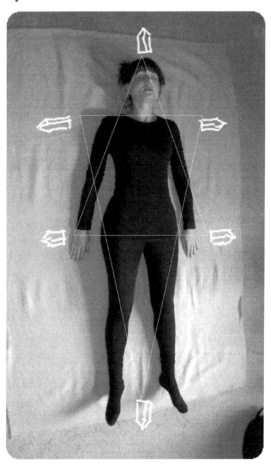

- To begin place all of the quartz crystals pointing outwards from the body.
- Make an upward pointing triangle using a point above the head and a point on each side of the hips.
- Make a downward pointing triangle using a point on the midline below the feet and a point either side of the shoulders.
- Imagine connecting the points up with lines of light to make the two interlocking triangles that create the Seal of Solomon.
- Allow 5-10 minutes of relaxation in the Seal of Solomon with the points facing outwards.
- Now turn all the points around so that they face inwards and allow a further 5-10 minutes of relaxation.

Variations

You can lengthen the amount of time spent in this layout, although you are unlikely to need more than half an hour for the complete treatment. You can use the Seal of Solomon around you when sitting up, whether cross legged on the floor, or sitting on a chair. You may also set up the Seal of Solomon around a body part in need of attention, such as hand or a foot.

You can use 6 matching tumblestones to expand the choice of crystal energies you have available. Tumbles won't direct the energy in the same way that points do however. Experiment with lying on different coloured cloths, look at the section on Colour in Crystal Healing for inspiration.

Touchstones
Clear quartz points: effective at transmitting pure white light.
Amethyst points: cleansing and deeply relaxing.
Smoky quartz points: increase feelings of protection and security.

Chapter Seven:
Crystals and the Chakras

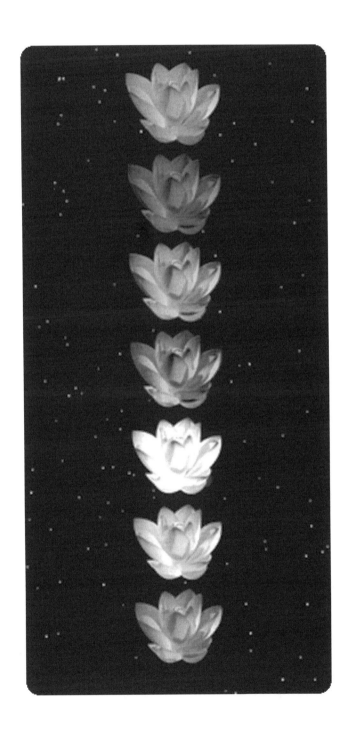

The Chakra System

Keeping your chakras healthy and functioning well will go a long way towards keeping you in great shape physically, emotionally, mentally and spiritually.

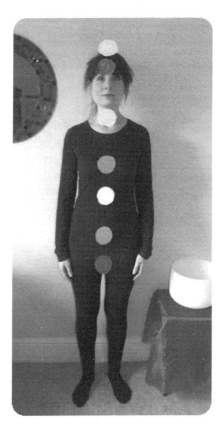

The main seven chakras are arranged along the spine and link in to the energy of the Sushumna, the central channel of energy that runs through the spinal column. This is the most important nadi, or channel of energy in the body and most people need to work on clearing this channel. Along each side of the Sushumna are two other nadis, Ida and Pingala, these intertwine and where they cross the chakras occur. Ida is the feminine, lunar current and it ends at the left nostril, Pingala is the masculine, solar current and it ends at the right nostril. There are said to be 72,000 nadis in the body, but these are the three most powerful currents.

Each of the chakras is traditionally depicted as having a specific number of petals and containing a symbol. This illustration below is the heart chakra showing 12 petals and containing the six pointed star, the symbol of perfect balance.

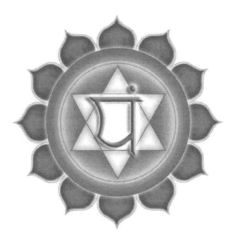

We all have our weaker and stronger chakras. Chakras may be overactive: too open, too full of energy, or spinning too fast. Chakras can be underactive: too small, clogged up, or spinning too sluggishly.

There are a range of opinions about which way the chakras should spin. In my experience healthy chakras normally spin clockwise, drawing energy inwards, however if they need to discharge excess energy they may spin anti-clockwise. It is important that chakras are neither stuck wide open, nor stuck closed. Your chakras need to be developed equally. Patterns where some chakras are wide open and over-active whilst others remain sluggish or closed can cause problems. You can gauge how open a chakra is and which way it is spinning by using a pendulum.

Bear in mind that none of the major chakras are more valuable than the others. People get confused by the terms 'higher' and 'lower' applied to the chakras; the Base chakra is every bit as important as the Crown! Their roles are distinct but equally vital. Your aim is to get all chakras cleared of debris, spinning freely and working in harmony.

When you start to focus on any one chakra you may find issues related to that chakra come to the surface. This may not be comfortable, but it is an opportunity to look at and clear things that may have been hampering the free flow of energy in your life.

The three 'Lower Chakras', the base, sacral and solar plexus, help us to handle life in the physical world and support us as raise our vibrational rate. Neglecting these three can create an unstable, ungrounded state and make it hard to cope with everyday challenges. Some spiritual seekers make the mistake of focussing most of their attention on developing the more 'glamorous' Brow and Crown chakras before creating the strong foundations necessary for spiritual growth. If you find you are becoming insecure or fearful, or simply unable to operate in the 'real world', then return to focus on the lower chakras.

My suggestions for crystals to support each chakra are only a guide; if you feel you need something else go with that feeling. I recommend you spend no more than 10-15 minutes at a time when you focus on an individual chakra. It is better to work little and often as the body can then assimilate the changes more easily.

The chakras which hold the most issues will need to be worked on over a period of time to clear and balance them. Be patient with progress!

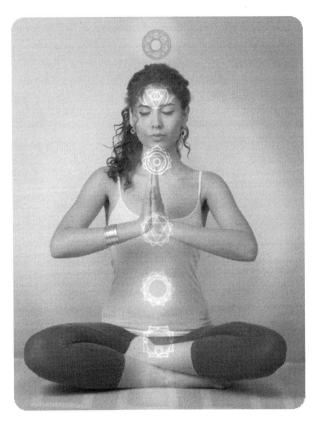

Should Chakras be Open or Closed?

Many spiritual healers and mediums believe that you should close your chakras when you 'aren't working'. Personally I think this is misleading as we are all meant to be using our chakras all the time. Chakras aren't just reserved for people leading a 'spiritual' life! However chakras can certainly be too open or too closed and you may want to consciously open them more fully when you are healing or in meditation and then close them down to a more modest size for everyday life.

If you are in good health your chakras will all be responsive. Imagine a sea anemone. Most of the time it is relaxed, openly taking in nourishment, but it will quickly withdraw into itself when it senses a threat, then when the danger has passed it opens out again. Ideally your chakras will open and close just as naturally. Unfortunately chakras are not always this responsive and they can sometimes get stuck in an overactive or tightly closed pattern.

Chakras are most often stuck open and overactive when someone has become addicted to the type of energy corresponding with that chakra area. Chakras can be kept tightly shut and underactive, or clogged up, when someone has experienced too much grief or pain in the corresponding area of their life. Closing down is a self protective response and a way of avoiding the issue rather than processing it; the associated energetic debris will need to clear before it can work healthily again.

A chakra that is stuck open or shut will have an impact on the corresponding area of that person's life. If a chakra is stuck wide open the person may be overwhelmed with too much information of that nature flooding into their system. If a chakra is stuck shut there will be too little.

One energetic pattern to be particularly aware of is the 'top heavy' pattern, where the crown and third eye chakras are overactive and wide open, but the lower chakras are closed and grounding is weak or non-existent. With the closing of the lower chakras there can be a disassociation from reality. In the healing world someone who is constantly tripping into the psychic realms without being well grounded and balanced in their lower chakras is often termed a 'space cadet' because their perceptions are all 'out there' but of little Earthly use. In extreme cases such a person can even appear to be quite insane, seeing and hearing psychic phenomena in an uncontrolled, overwhelming and indiscriminate way.

Simply channelling energy into an already overactive chakra will usually make things worse. The dominant chakras need calming down, underactive ones may need to be cleared or opened up. Sometimes it takes several balancing sessions before there is a noticeable shift in these patterns as the client can knowingly or unwittingly return their chakras to the pattern they have grown accustomed to.

Opening and Closing the Chakras

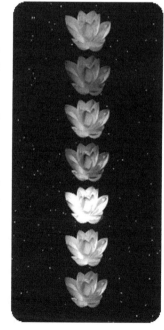

Sensitive people and those who suffer interrupted sleep may like to try closing their chakras at bedtime, but need to remember to open them again in the morning otherwise they will lack energy. Work from the base chakra upwards to open and the crown chakra downwards to close. This is a simple visualisation:

- Visualise each of your chakras as flowers that can open and close. You can add the typical colour of the chakra to your visualisation, so a red flower for the base, orange for the sacral, yellow for the solar plexus, green or pink for the heart, blue for the throat, indigo for the brow and violet, white or gold for the crown. Don't force these colours, you may perceive other shades.

- Picture each chakra as having petals that can be opened like a flower drinking in the sunshine and closed down again into a protective bud.

Chakra Attributes

Each chakra has a whole range of associations; I am only giving you a short summary over the following pages. Independent study of the chakras is recommended and some helpful resources are listed in the Further Study section.

Sanskrit names
Sanskrit is an ancient and sacred language and as far as I am aware it was through Sanskrit that the chakras were first described. The word *chakra* itself is Sanskrit meaning 'wheel' or 'disk'. The Sanskrit names are beautiful in their own right and reveal more of the nature of each chakra.

Colours
The colours listed are the rainbow spectrum colours used most frequently in the West. This system makes a lot of sense as working up the spine each chakra is of a higher vibration than the one below it, just as each colour of the rainbow carries a higher vibration as you move from red through to violet. There are however other colour associations for the chakras so don't feel obliged to follow this slavishly if something else feels more appropriate.

Elements
The first five chakras have an affinity with the elements in turn: Earth, Water, Fire, Air and Ether. Opinions vary over attributing elements for the Brow and Crown chakras.

Bija Mantras
These are Sanskrit 'seed sounds'. The sounds can be chanted to stimulate the chakras. Each chakra is traditionally depicted as a flower with a specific number of petals. If you enjoy chanting you can also use mantras to vibrate each petal of each chakra.

Endocrine Glands and Hormones
From a therapist's point of view understanding the correspondences between the chakras and the endocrine glands can give insight into a host of symptoms. The endocrines are ductless glands which secrete hormones into the physical system. There are over 50 different hormones controlling vital bodily functions such as your metabolic rate and sex drive. An imbalance in hormones can have very marked effects on your health; therefore supporting the endocrine glands by working on the related chakras can be an important part of restoring balance.

Senses
Each chakra has an associated sense organ.

Animals
Traditionally the chakras were associated with particular animals. It may be less obvious how to use this information in a literal way, but symbolically you could consider the animal and the way that it relates to the function of the chakra and you might want to focus on bringing those qualities into your life.

The Base Chakra
Sanskrit: Muladhara, meaning root support
Colour: Red
Element: Earth
Bija Mantra: LAM (*lahm*)
Endocrine gland: Adrenals
Main Hormones: Adrenaline, Noradrenaline
Sense: Smell
Animal: Elephant

Function
The base, or root chakra is our foundation for living and survival; it is located at the perineum. This is the chakra that helps us function within the physical planes of existence and acts as our anchor upon the Earth.

A healthy base chakra helps us keep our focus and be practical. Someone who needs to 'get real' probably has a dysfunction here.

The base is strongly affected by our childhood as it is our 'tribal' chakra. Here we find our sense of having 'roots' and belonging to a certain family, place or culture. If you had to move home or schools a lot as a child, or experienced insecure parenting your base chakra may need healing.

Physically it relates to our skeletal system, the underlying structure of our physical body. It is also the seat of passion at the immediate and instinctual level. The root chakra is linked to survival and the fight or flight response, controlled at a physical level by the adrenal glands.

The base chakra helps us to manifest ideas into reality; it anchors high spiritual energies so that we truly bring them into the world. A healthy base chakra can support us through times of change.

Signs of Dysfunction
Underactive: low energy, exhaustion, feelings of disassociation, unfocussed, lack of motivation, fearfulness, insecurity, loss of interest in physical world, feeling like you don't belong here.
Overactive: materialistic, bullying, selfishness, feeling indestructible and taking foolhardy risks.

Base Chakra Workout
Adopt a daily grounding routine
Eat healthy sustaining food
Take regular physical exercise such as walking or jogging
Take up gardening
Find healthy outlets for build-up of energy. Use a punchball or cushions if you need to work off aggression
Enjoy energetic passionate behaviour

Using Crystals to Support the Base Chakra
Choose one to four red crystals. Place them at or near the base chakra. Crystals can be placed between the tops of the thighs, let clients place the crystals for themselves, or place them one on each side of the chakra at the crease where the top of the legs meet the torso. Leave in place for five minutes and notice any sensations coming from the chakra. It may feel tingly, warm, or otherwise energised. Leave the stones for an extra five minutes if it feels right and then remove them.

Touchstones
Garnet: supports a sense of physical security in the world.
Ruby: stimulates a 'can do' attitude and a passionate love for life.
Red jasper: promotes physical stamina and strength.

The Sacral Chakra

Sanskrit: Svadhisthana meaning sweetness, or one's own place
Colour: Orange
Element: Water
Bija Mantra: VAM (*vahm*)
Endocrine Glands: Ovaries and testes
Main Hormones: Oestrogen and progesterone in women, testosterone in men
Sense: Taste
Animal: Crocodile

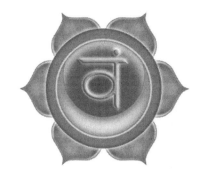

Function

The sacral chakra is associated with sensuality, creativity and magnetism. It is located below the navel. This is the place where deep-seated emotions are found, feelings about self-esteem and self-worth.

When the energy flows harmoniously here we are receptive to the pleasures of our earthly existence. This is the chakra of one on one relationships. Here we can build mutually supportive relationships with good boundaries.

The sacral is our centre of our creativity, whether that is the creation of new life in the womb, the crafting of a piece of art, or the baking of a cake. Creation is a sacred activity and it is no accident that 'sacral' and 'sacred' share the same origin. All humans have a need to express themselves through their creations.

The sacral chakra relates to the bladder, uterus and intestines. Its action is about 'letting go and letting flow', therefore any issue that indicates a lack of flow, whether that is manifesting at the physical level or not, could be linked to the sacral chakra.

Signs of Dysfunction

Underactive: lower back pain, digestive problems such as IBS, constipation, prostate and bladder problems, sexual dysfunction, menstrual issues, feeling guilty or ashamed.
Overactive: digestive problems such as IBS, diarrhoea, menstrual cramps, cystitis, jealousy, addictions, emotional volatility.

Sacral Chakra Workout

Ensure you have good levels of hydration, especially drink water
Take flowing exercise such as belly dancing, swimming, or tai chi
Take up creative pursuits including art, sculpture, crafting, knitting or sewing
Have fun, do things that will give you a 'belly laugh'
Have an aromatherapy massage
Enjoy a truly sensual personal life

Using Crystals to Support the Sacral Chakra

Choose between one and six orange crystals and place them on the lower belly. Leave the stones in place for five minutes and notice any sensations, perhaps warmth or tingling. There may be emotions welling up or emotional memories. Don't suppress these, let them flow and if tears come allow them. Leave the stones for an extra five minutes if it feels right and then remove them.

Touchstones
Carnelian: instils courage and promotes the confidence to take action.
Sunstone: warms and inspires, supports a healthy sex drive.
Fire agate: ignites passion and stokes the fires of creativity.

The Solar Plexus Chakra

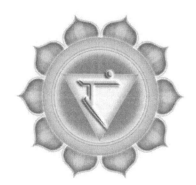

Sanskrit: Manipura, meaning lustrous gem
Colour: Yellow
Element: Fire
Bija Mantra: RAM (*rahm*)
Endocrine gland: Pancreas
Main hormones: insulin, glucagon
Sense: Sight
Animal: Ram

Function

The solar plexus chakra is the powerhouse where energy is transformed for use by the body, located in the centre of the body between the navel and the diaphragm. The energy generated here fuels the body and enables us to creatively take control of our lives. When the solar plexus chakra is working well we feel empowered and confident.

Some people confuse being empowered with having control over others. Historically this urge to dominate has led to dictatorships, wars and power being held over the masses. We need a new style of leadership where just decisions are made for the good of all. An empowered person with a healthy solar plexus can use their will with integrity.

A healthy solar plexus chakra supports our learning and absorption of new materials. It helps us think clearly for ourselves and to act assertively. Physically it influences the nervous system, the immune system and the digestive system.

Signs of Dysfunction

Underactive: insecurities, fear, powerlessness, self criticism, poor memory and learning, inability to make decisions, poor boundaries, poor absorption of vitamins and minerals.
Overactive: stomach ulcers and digestive disorders, auto-immune disorders, allergies, neuroses, 'knee jerk' decision making, domineering, controlling, overpowering behaviour, over competitiveness, judgmentalism.

Solar Plexus Chakra Workout

Pursue hobbies that interest you.
Keep a regular journal.
Learn to accept and appreciate yourself with all of your idiosyncrasies.
Try writing 10 things that you like about yourself each day.
Follow your 'gut instincts' and notice how your life runs when you pay attention to these.
Live with integrity; lying and half truths damage your sense of self-worth.
Try to show the same level of integrity in your dealings with people as you'd hope to be shown yourself.

Using Crystals to Support the Solar Plexus Chakra

Choose between one and ten yellow crystals and arrange them on and around the centre of your abdomen, the area below the diaphragm and above the navel. Leave the stones in place for five minutes. Pay attention to how the solar plexus is feeling. Attention may be given to feelings of empowerment. Notice where you give your power away. If appropriate leave the stones in place for an additional five minutes.

Touchstones
Citrine: inspires positive thinking, clarity of mind and strengthens the will.
Honey calcite: melts away old inhibiting patterns to reveal true motivations.
Yellow opal: bottled sunshine in a stone, an antidote to dull days, brightens the mood.

The Heart Chakra

Sanskrit: Anahata meaning unstruck
Colour: Green (also pink)
Element: Air
Bija Mantra: YAM (*yahm*)
Endocrine gland: Thymus
Main hormones: Thymus stimulating hormones
Sense: Touch
Animal: Antelope

Function

The heart chakra is the midpoint of the major chakras linking the lower and higher centres of the energy body. As such the heart chakra is the focus of emotional, physical, mental and spiritual balance, both within ourselves and in our relationships with others and the outside world.

The heart chakra governs the organs of the body that have actions of expansion and contraction, including the physical heart and the lungs. The work of the arms and hands is also closely linked to the heart chakra; think of the way arms encircle a dear one or push away something unwanted.

Emotionally the heart governs our loving relationships and is particularly active in relationships where there is unconditional love, such as a parent might feel for a child. When we fall in love we are experiencing heart chakra energy, whereas sexual urges have more to do with the sacral chakra.

When we have a balanced heart chakra we feel self acceptance and acceptance of others. We can forgive others. We live by our own values rather than blindly following the value systems laid down by family, religion or society. You 'follow your heart'.

Signs of Dysfunction

Underactive: low self-esteem, lack of concern, boundary issues, respiratory, circulatory and heart disorders, low immunity.
Overactive: overwhelming sense of responsibility for others, conditional behaviour, manipulative behaviour, boundary issues, respiratory, circulatory and heart disorders.

Heart Chakra Workout

Look at yourself in the mirror and love the person whom you see there. If you find this hard start with looking deep into your own eyes.
Look for the good in yourself and other people. Open your heart to become more accepting and forgiving; no-one is perfect.
Tapping in: Tap the breast bone in the centre of your chest several times with your fingertips. Tapping here helps to centre your energies and stimulates the thymus.
Make physical contact; enjoy a hug or stroke a pet. Pets are a source of unconditional love.

Using Crystals to Support the Heart Chakra

Choose between one and six pink or green stones. Arrange the crystals on or around your heart chakra at the centre of the chest. Leave them in place for five minutes. Notice how the heart chakra is feeling, it may feel warm and expanded or cold and contracted. Allow any bitterness, disappointments and heartache to be released. The stones can be left for a further 5 minutes if it feels right. People can hold a lot of pain in their hearts and it can take time and regular work to release this.

Rose quartz is a powerful heart healer. Hold it to your heart, allowing any bitterness, disappointments and hard-heartedness to flow into the stone. Cleanse the stone carefully and charge it between sessions.

Touchstones

Rose quartz: releases old hurts and promotes loving feelings and compassion.
Rhodocrosite: heals old wounds and promotes self worth and empathy.
Aventurine: soothes troubled emotions and brings new hope.

The Throat Chakra

Sanskrit: Vishuddha meaning purification
Colour: Blue
Element: Akasha / Ether
Bija Mantra: Ham (*hahm*)
Endocrine Glands: Thyroid and parathyroid
Main hormone: Thyroxine
Sense: Hearing
Animal: Bull

Function

The throat chakra is located at the base of the neck. Its prime function is communication and self-expression. If balanced you can speak your truth and express your self-identity and needs. You will be able to listen to others and empower them. You will be able to hear the truth in what someone is trying to communicate and so will not be prone to misunderstandings. A well functioning throat chakra gives a sense of peace and calm.

Physically the throat lets energy move through it; think of the passage of air, food and drink. It acts like a pressure valve, releasing build up in other chakras too. Expressing yourself or suppressing your thoughts and feelings will have knock on effects elsewhere too.

Signs of Dysfunction

Underactive: inability to speak up for oneself, loss of voice, stiff neck, shoulders, upper back pain, sore throat, headaches, isolation, emotional withdrawal, asthma, underactive thyroid.

Overactive: over verbose, speaking but not listening, agitation, lying, manipulation, dominance, shouting, overactive thyroid.

Throat Chakra Workout

Make some noise with your vocal chords, preferably harmonious, but not necessarily.
Try singing, it doesn't matter if you don't consider yourself a singer, do it anyway.
Chanting opens the throat chakra. The sound for the throat is 'ham' sounded *hahm*.
Honesty is good for the throat chakra. Speak your truth.
Check the language you use. When you talk do you tend to be upbeat or to moan?
Check what you are listening to. Uplifting messages, or spiteful gossip and human misery?

Using Crystals to Support the Throat Chakra

Choose between one and three blue crystals for the throat. Place them in the hollow at the base of the neck or on either side of the neck. Leave in place for five minutes. Notice any sensations. Notice what thoughts arise, especially note any situations where self expression has been stifled. If appropriate leave the stones for a further five minutes.

You may want to try making a gem water. Simply add spring water to a jug with a non toxic blue crystal such as blue lace agate. Allow the crystalline energies to permeate the water for an hour or more before pouring a glass and drinking. You can top up the jug with more water through the day. Keep the stone safely in the jug!

Touchstones

Blue lace agate: promotes harmonious expression of personal truth.
Angelite: envelops the user in peace and gently supports self-expression.
Aquamarine: cools and cleanses, promoting clear communication.

The Brow Chakra

Sanskrit: Ajna meaning to know or to command
Colour: Indigo
Bija Mantra: Aum (*ohm*)
Element: Light
Endocrine gland: Pituitary and Pineal gland
Main Hormones: Hormones that stimulate or
inhibit hormonal production by the other endocrine
glands from the pituitary, melatonin from the
pineal.
Sense: Sixth sense
Animal: None

Function

Also known as the 'third eye', this chakra enables us perceive and understand the world around us. It is located immediately above and between the eyes. As we travel on our spiritual path we do our inner work and gain 'insight'.

Well balanced the brow chakra can allow you to perceive from a state of detachment, not getting sucked into the emotional drama of a situation. You can be receptive and open to intuitive knowledge. Daydreams, dreams and visions are not bound by physical rules and can give us an enriched understanding and insight into ourselves and our world. Some people visualise in glorious 'Technicolor', whereas other people's mental images are more of an impression than a clear picture. This is still valid. If you are not naturally visual bring in more of the other senses to your visualisations, imagine the sounds, smells and sensations as well as the sights.

Most sources state that the endocrine gland associated with the brow chakra is the pituitary gland, however I believe the brow chakra is also related to the pineal as this gland is light sensitive as befitting the third eye. The pineal gland produces melatonin in darkness. This hormone makes us sleepy, so in Winter months we naturally feel more sluggish and in Summer more active.

On a physical level the brow chakra is related to the eyes, ears and nose.

Signs of Dysfunction

Underactive: depression, confusion, headaches, close-mindedness, lack of imagination.
Overactive: insomnia, nightmares, mania, headaches, delusions and hallucinations.

Brow Chakra Workout

Use creative visualisation. Imagine a beautiful scene, such as a lake, a forest, or a garden, in as much detail as possible.
Daydreaming is good for the third eye. Reverie is relaxing. Inspiration and solutions can come more easily when the mind's eye rests peacefully on a situation.
Imaginative and creative pursuits such as drawing, painting, writing and crafts exercise your third eye as you imagine the end result in your mind and work towards your vision.
Note your dreams. Dream images are often symbolic and need decoding. Their meaning sometimes needs reflecting on and can take a while to emerge.
Keep an attitude of open mindedness. Although you need to develop discernment it is helpful to be open to 'the possibility of possibility'.

Using Crystals

Choose one or two deep blue crystals to place on the third eye, above and between the physical eyes on the forehead. Leave in place for five minutes. Relax and notice sensations or images. Do not try and force the third eye open, just be relaxed with it. Allow an additional five minutes if it seems appropriate.

Touchstones

Lapis lazuli: helps one access deep wisdom and absorb profound teachings.
Azurite: supports insight and discernment, seeing what is beneath the surface.
Sodalite: aids clarity of perception and deepens intuition.

The Crown Chakra
Sanskrit: Sahasrara, meaning thousandfold
Colour Violet, Gold or White
Bija Mantra: Silent Om
Element: Thought
Endocrine Gland: Pineal gland, Pituitary gland
Main hormones: Melatonin from the pineal,
Hormones that stimulate or inhibit hormonal
production by the other endocrine glands from the
pituitary.
Sense: Beyond Self
Animal: None

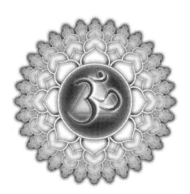

Function
The crown chakra is located just above the crown of the head. Here our consciousness can connect to the wisdom of our Higher Self, that part of us which is always in harmony with the Divine. Through a healthy crown chakra we may achieve a sense of Oneness with all Creation. The crown chakra opens us to the flow of Universal energy and it is through the crown that we receive healing energy for ourselves and for transmission to others.

If your crown chakra is working effectively you can expect synchronicity to occur with frequency. We experience a feeling of being peaceful, in tune with life and we feel guided to make wise choices. We are receptive to Divine inspiration and life feels meaningful and purposeful.

Most modern sources associate the crown chakra with the pineal gland. Although I think there is a link between the flow of Divine Light through the crown chakra and the pineal I sense that there is also an association with the pituitary gland which is often termed the 'master gland' as it controls the function of the other endocrine glands.

Signs of Dysfunction
Underactive: mental confusion, giving up, spiritually unaware, a 'what's the point?' attitude to life, headaches, feeling alone and separated.
Overactive: obsession, paranoia, agitation, irrational thinking, headaches, insomnia, messiah complex

Crown Chakra workout
Establish a daily spiritual practice.
Meditation
Contemplation
Communion with the Divine through prayer.
Practice gratitude for all the good you receive. There's always something to be grateful for.
Peaceful thoughts align you with your Higher Self.

Using Crystals to Support the Crown Chakra
Choose between one and five purple or clear crystals and place them in an arc just above the top of the head. If they are terminated then place the points facing outwards to relieve tension, or inwards to invite inspiration. Leave the stones for five minutes. Relax and notice any sensations, messages, impressions or inspirations. Leave the stones in place for a further five minutes if it feels appropriate.

Touchstones
Amethyst: stimulates intuition and connection with the Divine.
Charoite: aligns the self with a path of spiritual service.
Danburite: dissolves worries and fears, bringing joy and playfulness.

Photocopy friendly

Chakra Self Assessment

You can assess the state of your chakras by allowing an impression of each one to arise in your mind's eye in turn. What colour is it? How open or closed is it? Does it have a texture? Draw and colour each chakra on the chart. Large chakras may overlap the lines and small ones will not fill the circles. Over time your chakras can change so repeat this exercise and monitor your progress.

Name: **Date:**

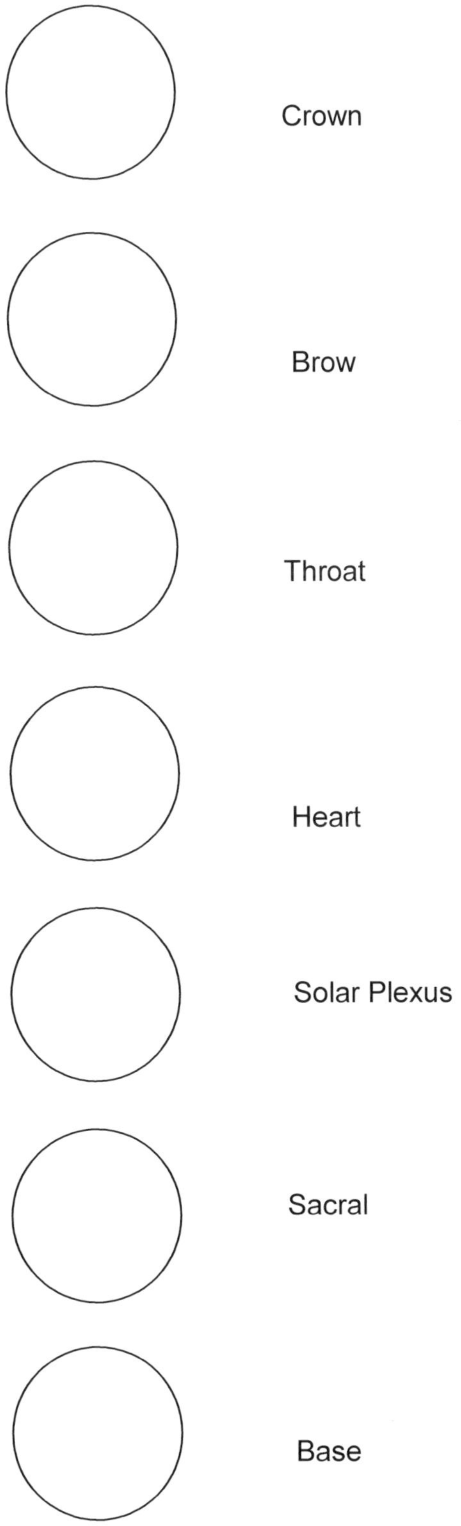
Crown
Brow
Throat
Heart
Solar Plexus
Sacral
Base

A Simple Rainbow Chakra Array

Although you can do a lot of good by working with one chakra at a time it is worth remembering that the chakras need to work harmoniously together as a team. Lying in a full chakra array is a very useful exercise and may be done once or twice a week. Remember healing often happens in layers, so that as you clear one issue another may bring itself to the surface for healing and release.

Method
Ensure you are energetically prepared to do healing.
Select a rainbow spectrum of crystals, one for each chakra:

Crown: violet

Brow: indigo

Throat: blue

Heart: green

Solar plexus: yellow

Sacral: orange

Base: red

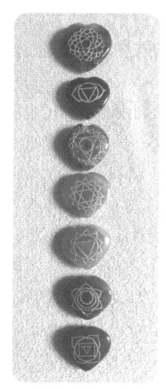

Add a grounding stone: usually black or brown

You can use this layout for yourself or a client. It isn't as fine tuned as other chakra balancing techniques, however it is straightforward and easy to perform.

- Place the grounding stone between and below the feet.
- Place each stone onto the corresponding chakra, starting with the base chakra and working up to the crown. If you are working on your own chakras have the selected stones to hand next to you when you lie down and then place them onto the chakras.
- Relax for five to ten minutes sensing how each chakra feels.
- When you are ready remove the chakra stones from crown down to base.
- Leave the grounding stone in place for a minute longer imagining grounding roots reaching deep into the Earth.
- When you are ready sit up and have a drink of water.
- Make a note of any impressions in your journal.

Assessing Chakras with a Pendulum

Chakras can be too open, too closed, too fast, too slow, swinging clockwise or anti-clockwise, blocked, chaotic or still. Healthy chakras will have a circular spin, will be moderately sized and usually clockwise in motion. Checking the spin of chakras with a pendulum helps you to spot any that are much bigger or smaller than the others, or much faster or slower. The aim is for the main seven chakras to all be spinning harmoniously together as a set, so that no one chakra is dominant and all are contributing to the whole.

By holding a pendulum over your client's chakras you can make an assessment of the spin. There is a front and rear aspect to each chakra other than the base and the crown. Front and rear aspects can be quite different from each other. Rather than turning your client over and disturbing their relaxation simply intend that you will be shown the rear aspect after you've assessed the front one. Be aware that when you begin dowsing your pendulum action can be over cautious and show the chakras as too small, or be wildly enthusiastic and show them as too big, so intend that you will be shown the true action of each chakra and try to relax. Assessing the chakras gets easier with practice.

Chakra Notation

I use a modified form of the chakra notation Barbara Brennan describes in Hands of Light. Using symbols like this saves a lot of writing and description on your client notes. Draw big symbols to show larger chakras and smaller ones for smaller chakras.

Here are the most common patterns you will encounter:

 Spinning clockwise and drawing energy in. Healthy pattern.

 Spinning anti-clockwise and sending energy out. Perhaps needs to release old energy for a while, but may need healing.

 Horizontal swing. Blocked. Not wanting to address an issue. Needs healing.

 Vertical swing. Blocked. Usually trying to avoid issue by attaching to the spiritual. Needs healing.

Still point. Chakra not moving. Needs healing.

Assessed Chakra Balancing

This method is easier to perform on another person, although you can ask your pendulum to show you the pattern of each of your own chakras by placing your free hand over the chakra in question and then choosing appropriate stones and laying them on yourself. An assessed chakra balance should be more precise than the simple rainbow array. Make each of your crystal choices with an intention of 'balancing the chakras'.

- Check you are ready to heal; if not sort your energies out before proceeding.
- Make sure your client is lying down comfortably.
- Assess the state of each chakra using your pendulum by holding it in the chakra energy. Remember there are front and back aspects to all but the base and crown chakras. Make a note of the pendulum swing for each one.
- Place a grounding stone or stones at one or more of the grounding points, see Grounding with Crystals.
- Starting from the base chakra and working upwards choose crystals with the intention to balance each chakra that needs healing and place them on the chakras.
- Check whether you need to add extra stones to any of the chakras and do so if necessary.
- Assess whether some additional healing energy is needed for any of the chakras. If so direct healing energy by channelling healing energy from your hand, or through a hand held quartz point into the chakras that need it.
- Stand back and wait until the crystals have done their work. This may be just a few minutes and it is usually no longer than 10-15 minutes.
- Remove the crystals when each chakra is balanced. Check the chakras individually as some may be ready before others.
- Keep checking until all the chakras are balanced.
- If this is the end of the treatment session then recheck grounding. Sit your client up and offer a drink of water.

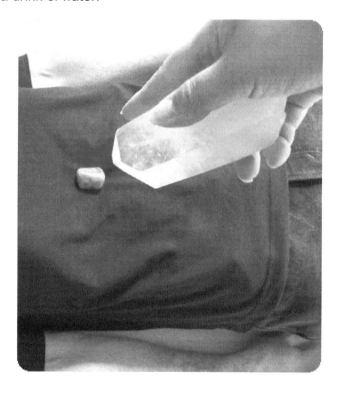

Releasing Congestion or Stimulating Chakras with Quartz Points

When you come across a chakra with a small or weak spin, or a chakra that feels clogged full of stuck energy you can help to restore balance using 4-6 smallish quartz points.

Where the energy seems blocked place the points evenly around a chakra balancing stone with the points directed outwards to release the stuck energies.

Where a chakra is lacking in energy place the quartz points evenly around the chakra balancing stone with the points directed inwards towards the chakra to bring fresh energy in. This is also helpful following the release of stuck energies to revitalise the chakra.

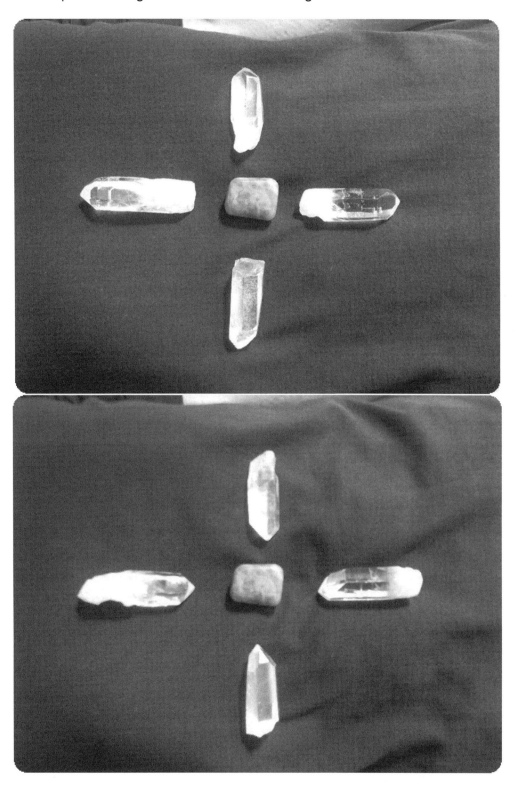

Photocopy friendly

Chakra Balance Record Sheet

Name: **Date:**

Chakra	Front aspect	Rear aspect	Crystal/s
Crown			
Brow			
Throat			
Heart			
Solar Plexus			
Sacral			
Base			
Grounding			

Any recommendations:

Chapter Eight:
Crystals and the Aura

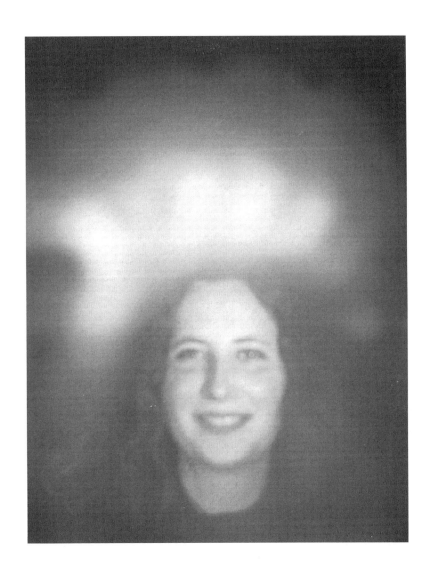

The Aura

When we refer to the aura we are talking about the energy field which surrounds the body. This is the energy that delineates your personal space and should be egg shaped and about an arm's reach all around you. Psychologists generally do not acknowledge the aura, but they do agree that we feel uncomfortable if someone we do not know well, or feel unsure about, comes into our personal space. I believe the reason for this is they are literally moving into our energy field. Someone with a strong, clear and vitalised aura will usually be in a good state of health. Someone with a weak, depleted and murky aura will usually not feel so good.

Empaths, who are often drawn into healing professions, need to take especial care of their aura as they have naturally sensitive boundaries that allow a lot of information from other people and the environment through. This can be helpful in the sense that you know how someone else is feeling, or whether a place has a good energy, however such sensitivity can also be quite tiring and the aura can take on board uncomfortable energies. Be particularly careful to keep your aura cleansed and your boundaries strong if this sounds like you.

Aura Awareness Visualisation

This visualisation heightens your awareness of your own energy field and helps you to maintain its integrity. You will need a clear quartz point and a piece of selenite.

Sit upright with your back free if possible and your feet flat on the floor. Take a few deep breaths. Take your awareness out into your aura.

Sense how far your aura extends from your physical body. Does it extend an equal distance all the way around you in a smooth egg shape? Could you touch the boundary with your arms outstretched? Does it bulge out further in some places? Is it closer in at one side or the other, or at the front or back? Does it extend under your feet and over your head equally?

Is your auric boundary good and strong all the way around or does it have some tears or holes? If so take the selenite and use it in a stroking movement to seal any rips or holes, and over any areas you feel are leaking energy. Keep smoothing over these places until you feel the boundary is secure again. If the damage is around your back or out of reach you could enlist a helper, or just visualise using the wand in that area.

Holding the quartz point in front of your face imagine each breath you take is quartz crystal energised and breathe that energy out into your aura focusing on any area that was too close to your body as if you are expanding a balloon. Draw any part of the aura that you felt was bulging too far away from you with your in breath. Keep working on your aura until you feel it is egg shaped, smooth, full of energy and within finger tips reach of your physical body.

Finally imagine a protective coating around the boundary of your aura, such as a crystalline shell. Bring your attention back to the contact your feet make with the floor, take a few deep breaths and open your eyes.

Touchstones
Selenite: seals and repairs holes and rips in the aura.
Clear quartz: revitalising, fills the aura with fresh energy.

Creating Healthy Auric Boundaries

You will need: 6-12 small clear quartz points, a crystal pendulum, a selenite wand

- Prepare yourself for healing. Your client may either be sitting in a chair or lying down. Sitting up makes it easier to check the aura at the front and back, whereas lying down allows you to check the extent of the aura below the feet and above the head. If the client seems to be ungrounded work on them lying down.
- Intend that you will be shown the boundary of the client's aura and walk slowly towards the client using your pendulum to feel the edge of the aura. It may swing to indicate the boundary, or you may sense the edge as a subtle resistance. You may also find you can sense the boundary through the palms of your hands. Place a quartz crystal as a marker on the floor to show the extent of the aura.
- Move around the client and sense where the edge of their aura is again, placing another quartz marker. Continue moving around the client in this way until you have made a complete circuit.
- Stand back and view the boundary. Most people with healthy auras keep them at about arm's reach. Is the auric boundary closer in or further out? Are there any places where the shape of the aura bulges out or dips in? Is it lopsided? The quartz outline should form a smooth egg shape around the client if they are lying down, or a smooth circle if they are sitting up, in both cases the client should be central in this.
- Intend that any adjustments you make will bring the boundary to the ideal place for your client at this time. Where the aura is bulging out too far turn the quartz markers to point inwards. Where the aura is dipping in turn the quartz markers to point outwards. Allow the directional energy of the quartz points to move the boundary.
- If required you can also encourage the aura to move by fanning it with your hands in the right direction.
- After five minutes recheck the position of the boundary with your pendulum. Move the points to the new position. Continue to move the points inwards or outwards until a smooth and even boundary has been established. Your client may sense the boundary moving and they may report warmth or tingling in the corresponding part of their body.
- When the boundary looks a healthy shape and size you can turn the points 90° to create a strengthening clockwise flow around the auric boundary.
- To check for any holes or tears in the aura pendulum dowse to ask whether any aura repairs are needed. If you get a yes response move your hand slowly around the auric boundaries, remembering that the aura is three dimensional. You may notice a chilly spot or a slight breeze which indicates leaking energy. This is a bit like a balloon with a slow puncture. Damage is often found at the back, therefore the client may need to turn over or sit up. Ask whether this is the case by dowsing.
- When you find a breezy or cold spot smooth over it with the selenite wand intending that the selenite will create an energetic shield over the hole which will seal it whilst the aura heals. Keep working in this way until the cold spot or breeze has gone. If the sensation does not diminish there may be another cause. Dowse whether you have done enough to seal the aura.
- I like to finish my crystal therapy treatments by sweeping a selenite wand over the aura with the intention that it will seal and protect the auric boundaries of my client.

Cleansing the Aura with a Pendulum

I learned this 'five line clearing' from Sue and Simon Lilly and it is a firm favourite with my students. It is simple and yet effective. Imagine that your client's body has five lines running vertically along it from head to foot. These are not actual energy lines, they are imaginary, used as guidelines in the treatment.

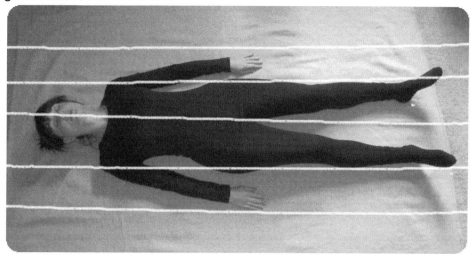

- First prepare yourself for healing.
- Stand at the feet of your client and put your pendulum into a neutral back forth swing. Set an intention that the pendulum will circle when you come across any dense energy in the aura which can be cleared quickly and safely with the pendulum.
- Now slowly move up the centre line of the body starting below the feet and swinging the pendulum across the line, pausing where the swing changes to a circular motion.
- Allow the pendulum to circle, stirring up the stagnant energy to clear it. Wait until the pendulum returns to its neutral swing. Continue to move up the centre line in this way until you finish above the head.
- Now repeat the process for lines 2 and 3 which can be visualised at about hip and shoulder width from the body. Start from the foot end each time. It doesn't matter which side of the body you do first, but keep things balanced by treating each side.
- Finally complete lines 4 and 5 which are about 1ft out from the body. If you are short of time you can finish at line 3.

Variations

You may prefer to keep the pendulum stationary as you move along each line, allowing it to circle when clearing the unhelpful energies. This allows you to sense any heavier energy as a resistance in the aura. Beginners may find this approach harder.

You can vary the healing with your choice of crystal pendulum and also by how high or low you hold the pendulum over the client. Holding it lower will clear the more physical layers of the aura, holding it higher will work on the more spiritual layers. Allow your intuition to guide you.

Touchstones

Clear quartz pendulum: brings clarifying white light to the aura.
Herkimer diamond pendulum: detoxifies the aura effectively.
Rose quartz pendulum: clears emotional baggage.
Citrine or rutilated quartz pendulum: lifts heavy thought patterns.
Lodestone pendulum: releases build up of Geopathic or electromagnetic stress.

Cleansing the Aura with a Massage Wand

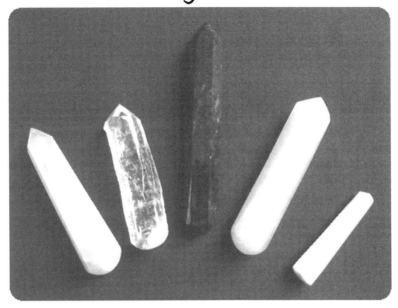

Crystal massage wands come in many types of crystal and different sizes. For this technique you'll need a wand shaped like those above, with a rounded base and a pointed tip. If you have several wands you can choose the most appropriate one for the client. Larger wands work on more of the aura at a time, however they will be heavier in your hand, so choose a wand that feels comfortable to hold.

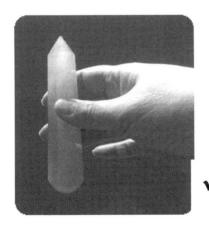

Hold the belly of the wand as shown here

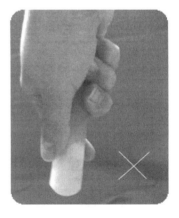

Do not cover the end with your hand when you are clearing heavy energies as you do not want to absorb these into your own system.

Touchstones

Clear quartz: clarifies the aura and fills with fresh energy.
Rose quartz: releases emotional hurts, infuses the aura with nurturing energy.
Smokey quartz: clears dense stagnant energies, fills the aura with protective energy.
Amethyst: purifies whilst calming, fills the aura with peaceful energy

Cleansing the Aura with a Massage Wand

This technique is easiest to use with the client lying down, but can be adapted for people who need to be treated in a chair.

- As always prepare your energy for healing.
- Stand to one side of the client at their feet holding the wand rounded end down. Keep the point facing upwards, not pointing towards you.
- Before you start set an intention that you will find and clear any stagnant energy from the aura that will be safe to remove at this time using the wand.
- Make anti-clockwise circular movements of the wand in the aura working across the body and slowly moving up the body from below the feet to above the head. You may vary the height at which you hold the wand and the size and speed of the circles you are making. Go with your intuition.
- You may find some areas feel 'thick' or 'sticky'. When you come to a dense area continue to work through it until it feels lighter or the wand moves more easily.
- If the wand starts to feel heavy in your hand imagine a bright golden bucket on the floor away from the client's energy field placed where you will not step in it. Give the wand a few sharp flicks into the bucket and you'll find it feels lighter again.
- Continue to work in anti-clockwise circles removing stagnant energy until you have covered the whole aura.
- Cleanse the wand again before turning it around in your hand with the point facing down.

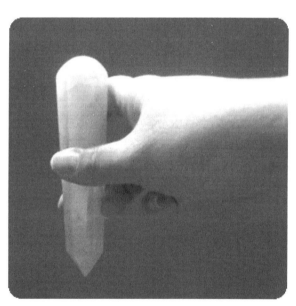

- Now make clockwise circular movements of the wand in the aura working back down the client from above the head to below the feet intending that you are replenishing the aura with fresh crystal energy. Again you may feel that in some places you need to slow down, speed up, make smaller or larger circles, or work higher or lower in the aura. Go with your intuition.
- Clear away the golden bucket of stagnant energy after your client has left. In your minds eye see it being lifted up by some helpers and taken off for transmutation.

The Subtle Bodies

The human energy field, or aura, is not one amorphous mass. It is made up of layers referred to as the subtle bodies which become progressively finer the further they are from the physical body. Each subtle body has a function. There are seven distinct layers to the aura and the functions relate to the chakras. You will find different names for the subtle bodies in some texts, I am using the terms I find most helpful. As we move outwards into the more spiritual layers of the aura it becomes much harder to find appropriate language to describe them.

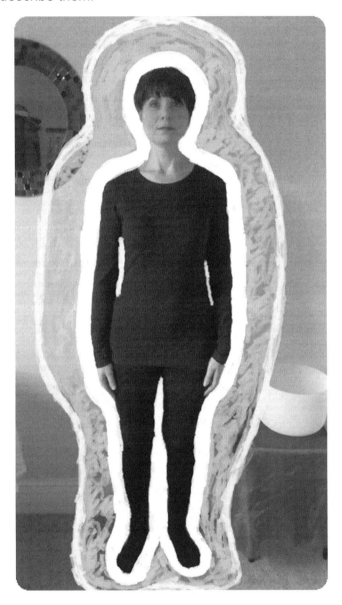

An impression of the first three layers of the aura. This is a cross section, remember the aura completely surrounds the body.

Most people can see the glow of the first layer, the etheric, which is just a couple of inches wide.

The second layer is wider, more nebulous and contains various colours which correspond to the person's overriding emotions.

The third layer is more structured and golden hued.

Few can visually perceive the individual subtle layers beyond, as they become increasingly fine and ethereal, however you can detect them with a pendulum and some people can locate them with their hands.

In 'Hands of Light' Barbara Brennan says the subtle bodies continue to alternate between structured and nebulous until the final structured layer of the Spiritual Body, which she perceives as golden threads of energy. For this reason visualising a golden boundary around the aura is strengthening.

The Etheric Body

The etheric body is the layer of the aura closest to the body. It is the easiest to sense as it has a slower vibration than the other subtle bodies. It can be best detected by gazing around the head and shoulders of someone against a plain white background in dim light. You may notice a glowing band around them, it is quite narrow, just an inch or so wide.

If you hold your hands out against a plain background you may see this band of energy and also 'etheric streamers' of energy coming from your fingertips. If you hold your hands with your fingers close together the energy will connect and merge and as you draw them apart it will stretch thinner, a bit like chewing gum, until eventually the connection is broken.

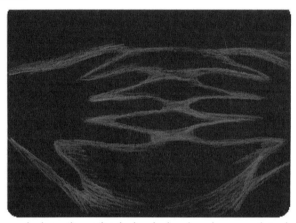

Like the base chakra, the etheric body is closely associated with the vitality of the physical body. For those who are old enough to remember the image of the 'Ready Brek kid' it is quite apt, although the etheric doesn't actually glow orange!

If the etheric is depleted and weak the physical body will lack energy. A healthy person with good energy levels will have an etheric body with a tangible `bounce' to it. You can feel the bounce of an energised etheric by sensitising your hands, as you would to choose a crystal, and then holding them an inch or two from someone. Avoid the main chakras as you'll start sensing those instead.

Kirlian photography visually captures some of the bio-electrical energy field emitted by living beings.

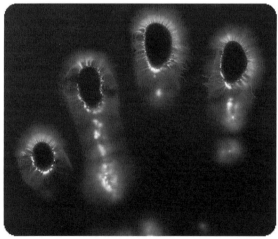

Touchstones
Clear quartz: supports physical energy levels.
Iron pyrites: boosts vitality and helps the body assimilate higher energies.
Red jasper: stabilises physical energies.

The Emotional Body

The emotional body is the next layer, relating to the sacral chakra. It is more nebulous than the etheric, composed of clouds of colour which respond to a person's moods and emotions. This is the layer that those who perceive auras as colours are most likely to be looking at. Seeing at this level comes easily to some people. You can try gazing at someone standing against a plain background and you may develop this ability over time and with patience. If you can't see anything with your physical eyes try looking with your mind's eye. What colour do you imagine the aura as?

The colours of this layer can change from moment to moment, but people do have a tendency to show certain colours, therefore a person who is often angry or aggressive is likely to display a lot of dark red in their emotional body, whereas someone who is on a healing path may have green. Generally bright clear colours are a sign of positive and healthy emotions, whereas murky, darker shades reflect unhealthy moods. Working in the emotional body can help to resolve emotional blocks.

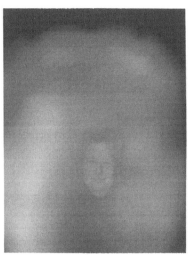

The aura photos you can have taken at Mind Body Spirit fairs seem to correspond most closely to the emotional body. I'm not sure how they work, but there does seem to be some correlation between your overriding emotional state and the resulting aura photo. The aura photo at the start of this chapter was taken immediately following a meditation. It was interesting to see how much bright white light stacked around my crown chakra when I had been communing with the Divine.

The photo here is my 'standard' aura. It is bright green over my head, blue on my left, gold on my right and purple in the middle. My aura has appeared this way again and again over the years. Aura colours do change according to mood. Once I had an photo taken when I was feeling a little harassed. I got a red, orange and yellow aura photo!

Touchstones
Rose quartz: provides nurturing, loving energy, enhancing self worth.
Moonstone: soothes and harmonises emotions to bring peace.
Aventurine: supports a more uplifted and positive outlook.

The Mental Body

The mental body is bright yellow and relates to the solar plexus chakra. It is more structured than the emotional body and becomes vibrant and expanded around the head when our thought processes are fully engaged.

Thoughts take shape, quite literally as thought forms in our aura. Thoughts are powerful, and the more habitual a thought is the stronger shape it will take, whether that is positive or negative. This is part of the reason that most older people tend to get very fixed in their opinions. It is hard to change someone's mind if they have held a belief for a long time, even if you can show it is erroneous. To change their thinking they need to dissolve the thought form related to that opinion. Working in the mental body can aid clear thinking and the release of old limiting thought patterns.

Touchstones
Citrine: supports a clearer, positive, more alert, state of mind.
Rose Quartz: encourages more loving and forgiving thought patterns.
Amber: dispels negative thought patterns and encourages positive thinking.

The Astral Body

The astral body is the fourth layer of the energy field, relating to the heart chakra. It appears to be similar to the emotional body but vibrates at a higher level and the colours have a more subtle, finer quality. It is the boundary between spiritual and physical energies. The astral is particularly active in our interrelationships with people. We test people out on an astral level to see if we will get on with them and send out welcoming or 'keep clear' vibes to others from this layer.

Touchstones

Moonstone: promotes tranquillity and ownership of feminine power.
Rose quartz: supports loving relationships and self worth.
Smokey quartz: assists in the creation of healthy relationship boundaries.

The Causal Body

The causal is the fifth level of the aura relating to the throat chakra. Its function is connected with our intention and when clarified it can support the understanding of and willingness to fulfil our life purpose. This is such a fine level that few detect it visually, however Barbara Brennan perceives this layer like an architect's drawing of clear lines on a cobalt blue background.

Touchstones

Lapis lazuli: helps in accessing deep inner knowledge and wisdom.
Clear quartz: promotes clarity of communication and thought.
Aqua aura: supports harmonious integration of higher energies.

The Soul Body

The soul body is the sixth layer of the aura, relating to the brow chakra. It is the highest emotional level raising us to a spiritual level of connectedness where we experience our Unity with and unconditional love for the rest of creation. Here we align with our Divine Self and experience unconditional love. It has a shimmering quality to the light which radiates out from it in iridescent beams.

Touchstones

Angel aura quartz: rainbow shimmers help one experience this fine level.
Rainbow moonstone: heavenly blue flashes of light assist Unity consciousness.
White precious opal: rainbow light supports integration of higher states of being.

The Spiritual Body

The spiritual body is the seventh layer of the aura which relates to the crown chakra. It is the finest layer of the aura. As the name suggests this level is where we know we are One with the Divine and indivisible from the Whole. To clairvoyant perception it appears as shimmering fine golden threads surrounding the egg shape of the aura and protecting the energy field with golden light. For this reason imagining your aura enclosed in a golden egg of light will strengthen the outer boundary of your aura.

Touchstones

Danburite: uplifts and promotes connection with higher realms of being.
Herkimer diamond: encourages integration of spiritual awareness into the physical.
Phenakite: carries a potent high vibration which can bring spiritual initiation.

Subtle Body Stone Placements

I was taught these stone placements by Sue and Simon Lilly and I have found them useful for treating specific subtle body layers. Often you will find that your client will benefit from a stone placement to a layer of the aura which corresponds to the chakra that needed most healing, although this isn't always the case.

You can use the Subtle Bodies Dowsing Arc or simply dowse by running your finger down the list below to determine which layer of the aura needs attention. The Touchstones I suggest for each layer are appropriate choices for these placements, but you may intuit others. The stone placement locations act as 'access points' to each subtle body. Check how many crystals are required and how long they need to be left in place. When the treatment is complete remove the stones and check whether any further work on the subtle bodies needs to take place. Just treat one subtle body at a time to avoid confusing the client's energies.

Subtle Body	Stone Placement	Suggested Stones*
Etheric body	No specific point. Dowse for best placement	Clear quartz Iron pyrites Red jasper
Emotional body	Stomach	Rose quartz Moonstone Aventurine
Mental body	Left hemisphere of the brain. Place the stone or stones around the left side of the head, checking correct placement of each.	Citrine Rose quartz Rutilated quartz Amber
Astral body	Kidneys. Check to see if different stones are needed near each kidney or whether the same type is needed on both sides. Tuck the stones under the back at about the level of the elbow.	Moonstone Rose quartz Smokey quartz
Causal body	Medulla Oblongata. Place in the hollow at base of skull. Use a smooth stone!	Lapis lazuli Clear quartz Aqua aura
Soul body	Pineal gland. Place at centre of forehead.	Angel aura Rainbow moonstone White precious opal
Spiritual body	Pituitary gland. Check for best placement: behind the head, level with the ears, behind the crown, or at the forehead.	Danburite Herkimer diamond Phenakite Azeztulite

*For the original list of suggested stones see Simon Lilly 'Illustrated Elements of Crystal Healing'.

Photocopy Friendly

Subtle Bodies Dowsing Arc

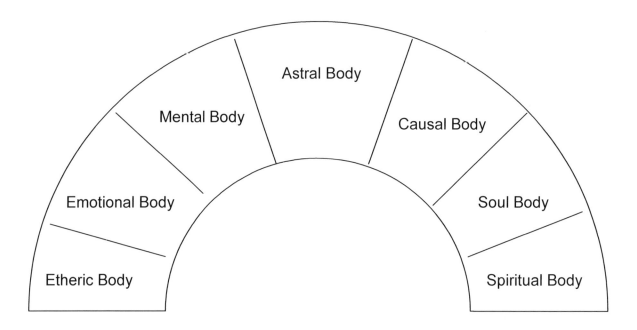

Chapter Nine:
Colour in Crystal Healing

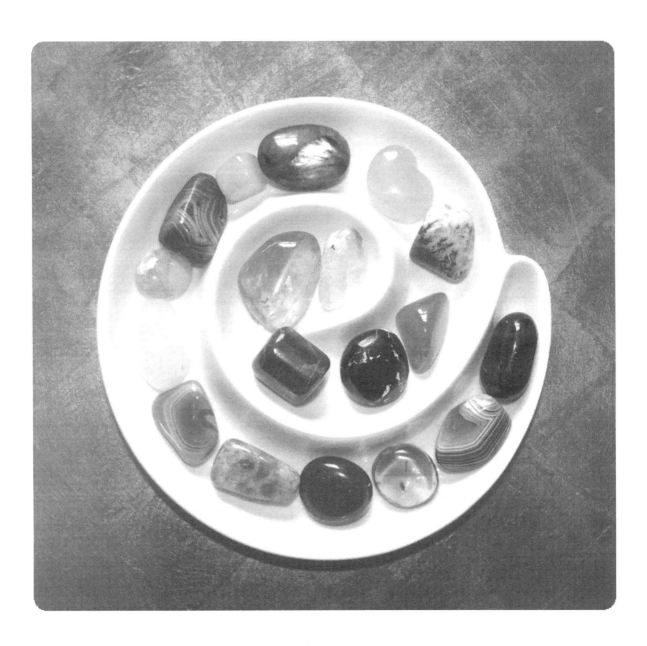

Using Colour in Crystal Healing

Colour is just one way in which crystal healing is thought to work. The basic rainbow chakra array simply matches the colour of crystals to the typical colours of the chakras to help bring them back to their correct vibration. An awareness of colour properties can help you understand some of the general properties of crystals in that colour range. Colour is also a very useful tool for visualisation and can be used for working on yourself as well as a client.

Colour is rich part of our lives; just think how depressing a monochrome world would look! The use of colour in our language can give us some clues about how colours affect us physically, emotionally, mentally and spiritually. Think about these phrases:

seeing red   feeling blue   rose tinted spectacles   going for gold

green with envy   grey around the gills   in the pink   whiter than white

Someone who is happy and in good health will show beautiful colours in their aura. Pastel and bright clear shades are usually positive, whereas dull, murky colours are an unhealthy sign denoting poor health or negative thoughts and emotions.

What is Colour?

Colour is light of different wavelengths and frequencies and light is just one form of energy made up from photons. We are all surrounded by electromagnetic waves of energy of which colour is only a very small part as you can see from the diagram below:

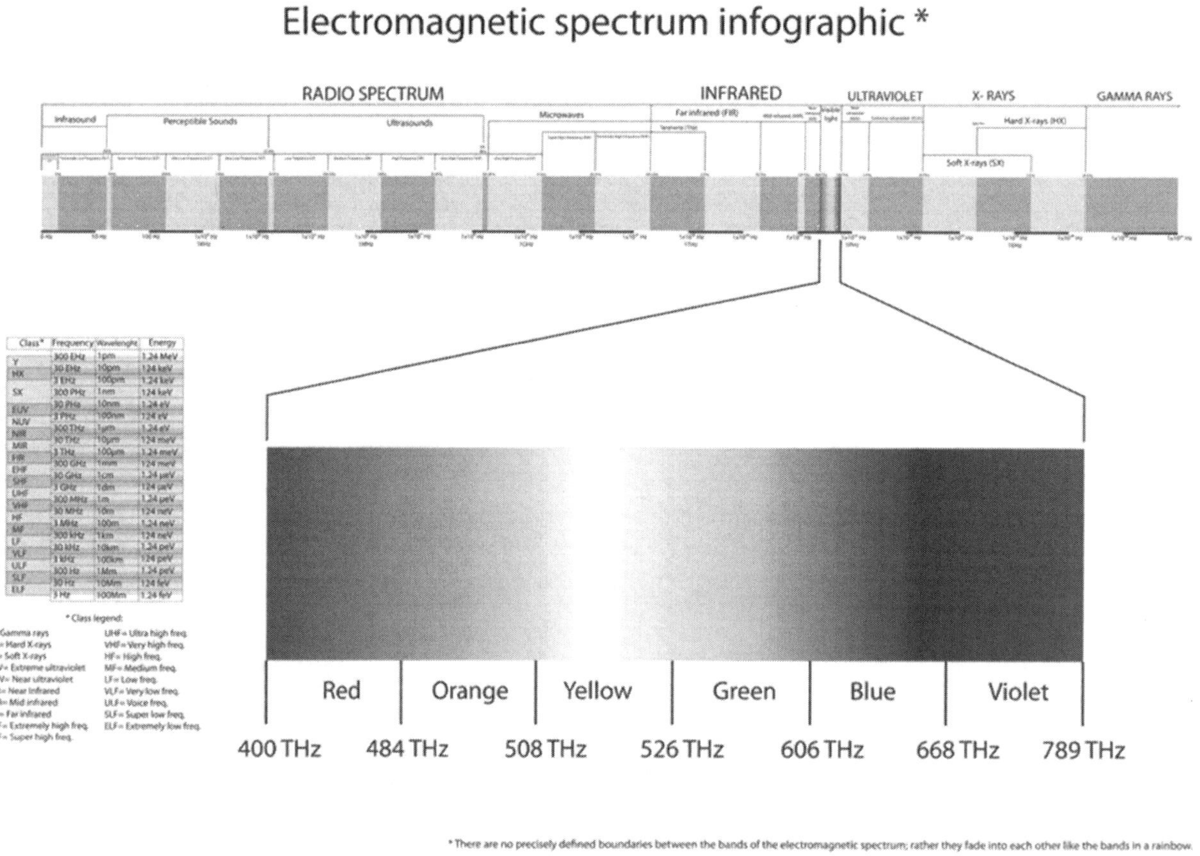

Electromagnetic spectrum infographic *

| Red | Orange | Yellow | Green | Blue | Violet |

400 THz   484 THz   508 THz   526 THz   606 THz   668 THz   789 THz

* There are no precisely defined boundaries between the bands of the electromagnetic spectrum; rather they fade into each other like the bands in a rainbow.

The visible spectrum as we see it consists of the rainbow. The seven colours of the rainbow spectrum all have different wavelengths and frequencies. Each colour is measured in units of cycles or waves per second. Red is at the lower end of the spectrum and has a longer wavelength and lower frequency contrasting with that of Violet at the top end of the spectrum which has a shorter wavelength and higher frequency.

White light is split into the full spectrum by a prism, which is what happens when the sun shines on raindrops and creates a rainbow.

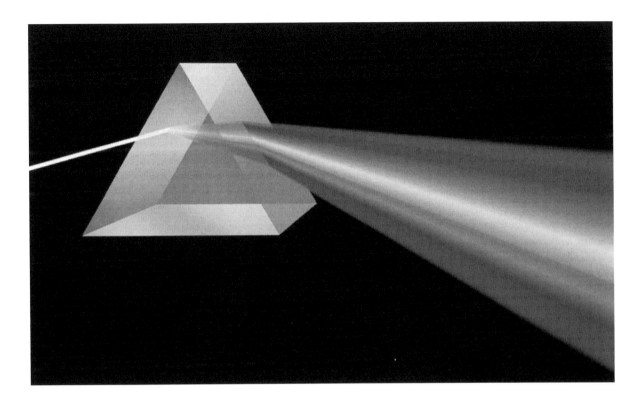

Red

Red is a warming colour. Clear, bright red in the aura is a sign of dynamism, vitality and energy. It is a colour associated with action. Most children will have lots of clear red in their aura. A predominance of darker red may indicate anger or even violent tendencies, hence 'to see red', this is more apparent as the red becomes darker and denser.

Used therapeutically red can balance the base chakra and boost energy levels and the immune system. Red can also aid muscular disorders. Red is not helpful where there is already an excess, whether that be emotions such as frustration or anger, or physical issues such as high blood pressure.

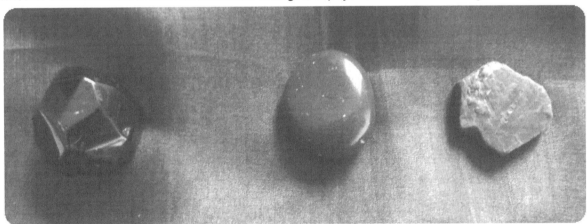

Touchstones

Garnet: fosters a confident, secure and assertive approach to life.
Red jasper: promotes inner strength and a down to earth practicality.
Ruby: encourages lust for life and enthusiasm, increases life force energy.

Orange

Orange in the aura denotes self esteem, confidence and a warm, joyful personality. As a combination of red and yellow it combines the properties of both to support thoughtful action. A dull orange can show egocentricity.

Therapeutically orange has many of the energising, warming, qualities of red without the risk of provoking anger. It is useful after a shock to promote fortitude and help restore equilibrium. Orange balances the sacral chakra and the reproductive system.

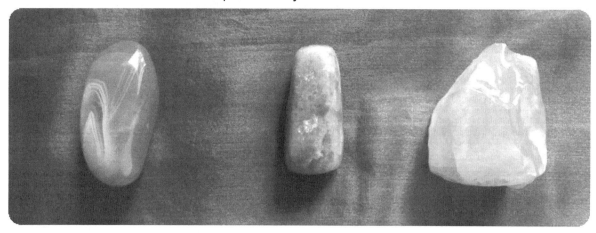

Touchstones

Carnelian: instils courage, strength and a creative response to life's challenges.
Sunstone: revitalises and uplifts, a warming energy reminiscent of the Sun.
Orange calcite: infuses the being with a gently playful and optimistic energy.

Yellow

Yellow in the aura shows someone who spends their time thinking and concentrating. Clear yellow is an uplifting colour. Dull yellow can show a possessive, jealous nature. Gold in the aura is very special and shows a highly spiritual person; think of the halo shown around the heads of saints.

Used therapeutically yellow is balancing for the solar plexus chakra and stimulates the metabolism. It is good for the digestive system, liver and kidneys. It is the most anti-depressant colour ray. Yellow can also support clear thinking, good at exam times!

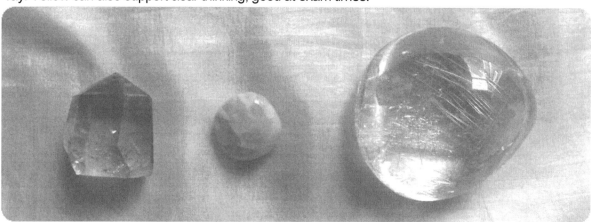

Touchstones

Citrine: promotes an optimistic outlook, aids concentration and study.
Yellow opal: supports a cheerful viewpoint, looks like bottled sunlight.
Rutilated quartz: sharpens thinking, encourages mental alignment with Divine Will.

Green

Green is a balanced colour occurring at the point between the lower vibrational warm colours and the higher vibrational cool colours. It is no co-incidence that green is the colour of the heart chakra. Green shows a loving energy and is associated with healing and energy from nature. Murky green shades such as khaki are unhealthy; hence 'green around the gills'.

Therapeutically green is a strong healing energy. It is good for heart and circulatory disorders. Green is not so helpful colour if growth is happening too fast as in eczema or psoriasis. Cooling colours such as blue are better choices if such a condition exists.

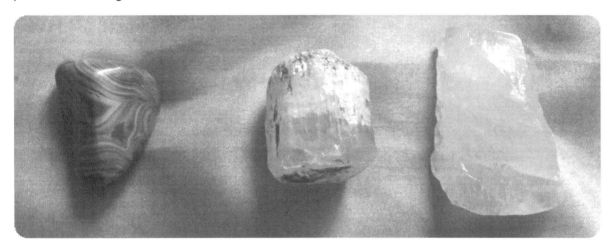

Touchstones
Malachite: absorbs and removes stuck emotions and heavy thought patterns.
Emerald: heals the emotions and opens the heart to accept love.
Green calcite: cools, like a balm for irritation, physical, mental or emotional.

Blue

Blue is the first of the cooling colours in the spectrum. Blue in the aura may show healing and psychic energy. Blue is a spiritual colour and symbolic of purity; think of the blue robe that the Virgin Mary is always depicted in. It clarifies the mind and gives a feeling of unboundedness, hence 'blue sky thinking'. In Buddhist philosophy blue is the colour of the clear mind.

Used therapeutically blue is cooling, calming and sedative. Good for balancing the throat chakra, sore throats, respiratory system and conditions where there is inflammation, angry or irritated energy.

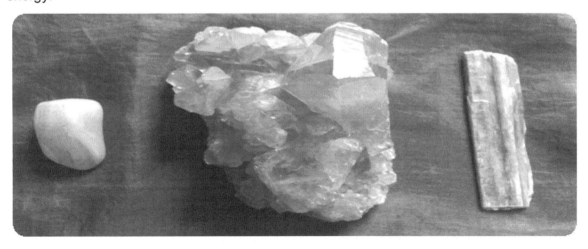

Touchstones
Blue lace agate: soothes and calms, helps one speak one's truth in a gentle way.
Celestite: inspires spaciousness, a heavenly blue stone with a peaceful vibration.
Kyanite: clears channels of communication and enhances positive connections.

Indigo

Indigo is associated with wisdom, depth and profound inspiration. It is a colour that supports inquiry within. In the aura it denotes a committed person with strong personal integrity. Too much indigo may suggest aloofness and detachment.

Therapeutically indigo is deeply calming. It can help to balance the brow chakra and may be used to gain deeper personal insight. Avoid indigo where the client has become too inward looking.

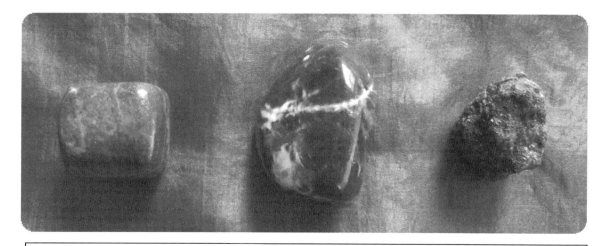

Touchstones
Lapis lazuli: strengthens the third eye, encourages one to look for wisdom within.
Sodalite: supports truth and integrity, an ally on the quest to 'Know Thyself'.
Azurite: promotes deeper perception and insight into hidden motivations.

Violet

Violet is deeply relaxing and encourages you to let go of everyday concerns. Violet in the aura shows a spiritual nature and highly developed consciousness. Excess violet can be a sign of escapism. As someone wisely commented, "You can't make a rainbow with just the colour purple."

Therapeutically violet can be used to help develop spiritual understanding and to balance the crown chakra. It can stimulate the imagination. Violet is soothing and sedative, so promotes sleep. The violet flame purifies and a violet cloak may be visualised to provide psychic protection.

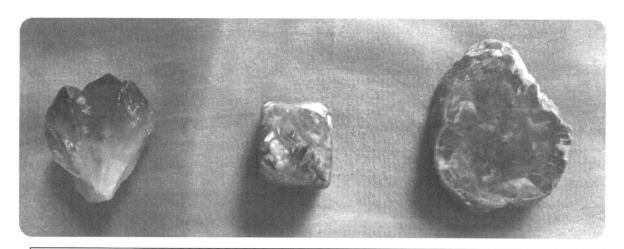

Touchstones
Amethyst: opens awareness of the spiritual and supports a peaceful outlook.
Charoite: assists in clearing old beliefs and attitudes that block spiritual progress.
Lepidolite: promotes deep, restful sleep, a tranquil, calming energy.

Violet marks the end of the rainbow spectrum, but there are other colours worth considering in crystal healing.

White or Clear

White is the colour formed by all the other colours of the rainbow. It is associated with purification, spiritual awareness and connection with higher energies. White provides a 'clean sheet' allowing you to start anew.

White light is considered the universal healer because it contains the whole spectrum. It can dispel heavy energies from the energy field and will fill the space with life force energy. Visualise white light shining from clear quartz crystals as you work with them, you may start to see the light emanating from the point.

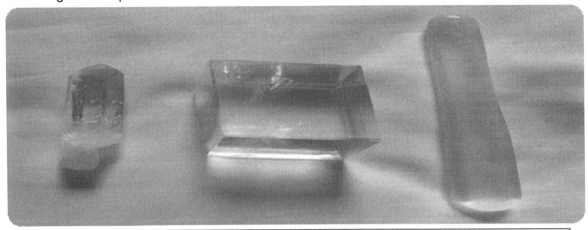

Touchstones
Clear quartz: carries the frequency of pure white light, the universal healer.
Selenite: purifies, sweeps away stagnant energy and brings light in.
Howlite: calms and quiets the mind, promotes peaceful sleep.

Black

Black is the Void from which all things come and it is rich with unmanifest potential. Without visual distraction in the darkness our thinking may become deeper and our other senses sharpen. Black is not a healthy colour in the aura, it shows stagnant, unhelpful energy.

Therapeutically black is very grounding and can also be used for protection. Notice how many teenagers turn to black clothing at this time of sensitive transition. Funereal clothes help the mourners cope with their loss. The overuse of black can lead to despondency and depression so use black in moderation.

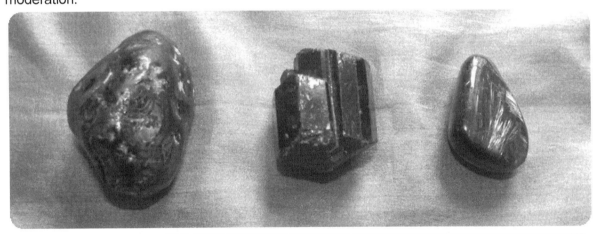

Touchstones
Apache tears: comforts in times of loss, supports the releasing of old grief.
Black tourmaline: grounds and protects strongly, alleviates insecurities.
Astrophyllite: allows one to simultaneously stay grounded and connect to the cosmos.

Turquoise

A colour ray of the New Age Turquoise connects the green of the heart with the blue of the throat allowing honest expression of the emotions. It evokes the calm beauty of a tropical lagoon.

Therapeutically this ray balances the higher heart chakra and brings freedom to be who you want to be rather than following the conditioning of parents, peers and society. It is an ally on the path to personal wholeness.

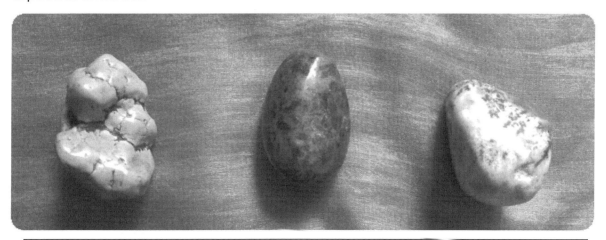

Touchstones
Turquoise: helps one speak what is in one's heart, a stone of truthful communication.
Chrysocolla: carries the energy of the Divine Feminine, instils reverence for Nature.
Larimar: cools and nurtures, bringing peace to troubled minds and emotions.

Pink

Pink in the aura shows a loving nature. When two people fall in love their auras will show a beautiful pink. This colour also reflects loving family relationships. Pink is the colour of the heart chakra of someone who has learnt to love unconditionally; needless to say most of us aren't quite there yet!

Therapeutically pink will help to heal the heart chakra, soothing a 'broken heart' and other heartfelt hurts. It can support someone in learning to love themselves as well as opening the heart to compassion for others.

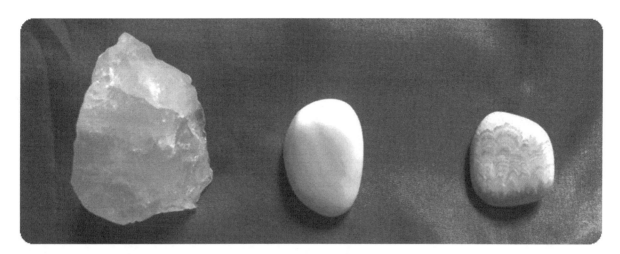

Touchstones
Rose quartz: heals old emotional wounds, the premier heart healing stone.
Mangano calcite: nurtures and comforts, one of the gentlest healing energies.
Rhodocrosite: transforms old emotional pain and low self worth, has a strong action.

Brown

Brown is a colour of the natural world reminding us of rich and fertile soil and the coats of many creatures which use brown to blend into the background. In the same way it can help us quietly to get on with our lives without drawing undue attention to ourselves. Brown isn't normally seen in a healthy aura. Too much brown can feel heavy and dull, so use in moderation.

Therapeutically brown is grounding and helps strengthen the connection to Earth energies. A practical and steadying influence, brown stabilises those prone to over dramatising. Brown is the best colour to bring a 'space cadet' back down to Planet Earth.

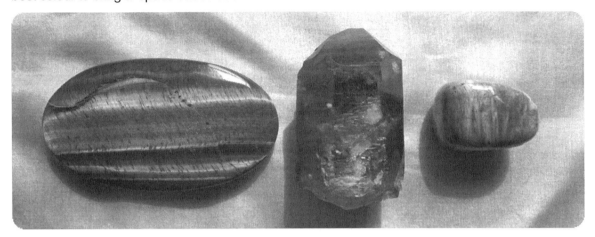

Touchstones

Tiger's eye: promotes feelings of security, self-assuredness and optimism.
Smoky quartz: gently grounds, protects and cleanses, stills mind chatter.
Petrified wood: stabilises and supports, whilst connecting to ones ancestral roots.

Grey

Grey is a quiet colour, think of the effect created when mist shrouds the landscape. Grey muffles and softens sharp edges. When worn as a business suit it masks the individual personality so that the wearer blends in.

Therapeutically grey is calming and can help soothe shattered nerves. It is a protective colour. Visualising yourself wrapped in a grey cloak can help you withdraw from the pressures of the world at stressful times. Use sparingly as too much grey can be depressing.

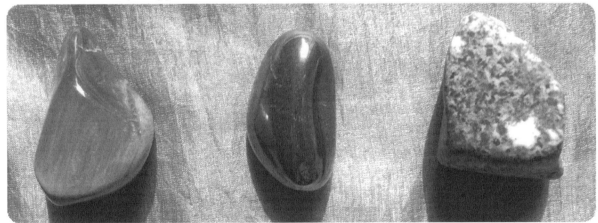

Touchstones

Tremolite: soothes the senses, peaceful, gives a sense of retreat.
Hematite: grounds strongly, anchoring the energy field firmly to the Earth.
Preseli bluestone: grounds, relaxes, evokes ancient British heritage.

Organising your Collection by Colour

Organising your stones by colour can be a simple way to locate the crystals you need. Tumblestones may be kept in bowls or bags together, providing you are gentle with them. Mine are kept on shelves in divided glass dishes to make selection quick and easy.

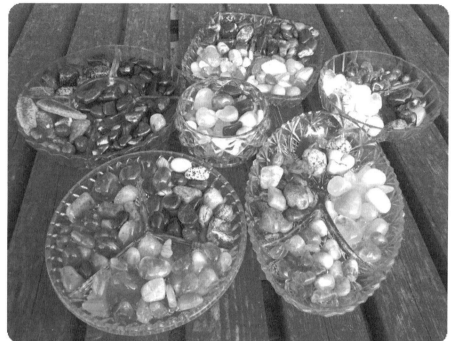

Crystal specimens need more careful individual storage to avoid damage. You can buy various segmented trays and boxes. I use a collector's cabinet. It has the advantage of protecting my crystals, but you can't see them without opening drawers. It helps that I group my crystals by colour and use the colour spectrum to organise the drawers. Prior to this investment I used open trays which were easy to cast one's eye over.

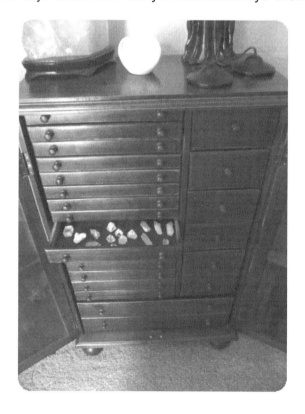

Photocopy Friendly:

Colour Dowsing Chart

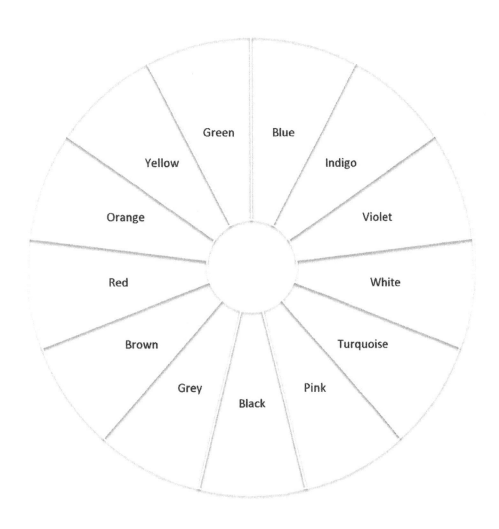

Healing with the Rainbow Spectrum

Whenever you use a crystal the colour will be significant, so it is worth bearing the colour associations in mind when you reflect on your crystal choices for a healing. You may consciously choose to apply crystals of a particular colour for your client and can intuit or use the Dowsing Chart to ascertain the most beneficial colours.

Crystal Nets

Crystal nets, or grids, combine colour and crystals perfectly together. Sue and Simon Lilly have been prolific 'crystal netters' and have published their nets in several books. Investing in a spectrum of cloths is worthwhile, I buy two metres of polycotton as it is easily machine washable and comes in a good range of colours, but you can use a white cloth if you don't have the right colour.

Guidelines for use

Nets are excellent for self treatment as well as for use in therapy sessions. Although simple to look at, crystal nets can be very powerful, therefore follow these guidelines:

- Allow plenty of time both for lying in the net and coming back to everyday consciousness.
- Make sure there will be no disturbances. Unplug or switch off phones.
- Lay the net out. If you don't have the right colour cloth then use a white one. For maximum benefit align the net with magnetic north at the head as this places the human energy field in alignment with the flow of the Earth's energy field.
- If you are the therapist stay very quiet whilst your client is in the net. Your role is to place the stones and keep an eye on the clock. You should be a reassuring presence in the room allowing the client to relax more deeply.
- There can be a deepening of experience approximately every five minutes. Best times to finish therefore are 5, 10, 15 or 20 minutes, as the client tends to surface a little in consciousness before sinking down to another level. You can check the time required by dowsing or intuit the time needed. I find I just 'know' when it is time to bring someone back out.
- Lying in a net for ten minutes several times a week is usually more therapeutic than one lengthy session.
- If there is any anxiety or discomfort the client can be told they may quietly come out of the net and relax for a while, before choosing whether to re-enter it or end that part of their treatment.
- Afterwards offer a drink of water and allow some quiet time to integrate the experience. Feelings or impressions should be noted soon after sitting up as the images and sensations can melt away quickly.
- As with any crystal treatment check grounding is in place before getting on with anything else.

The Amethyst Healing Net

This was the first net that Sue and Simon Lilly developed and it is very useful. Generally it is perceived as deeply relaxing and an aid to healing. Where there is an issue that needs insight the amethyst healing net provides a safe and protected space for deep enquiry and contemplation.

Requirements: Eight equally sized amethysts, preferably points. If two points are larger place one above head and one beneath the feet. Spread the rest evenly around the body. Points should face inwards. Lie on a violet cloth for relaxation, or yellow if uplifting is needed.

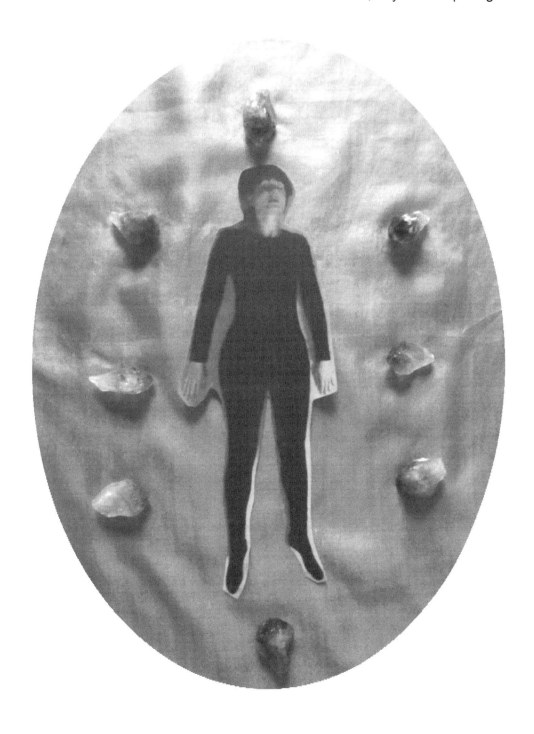

I give you the Sun, the Moon and the Stars

It is hard to attract good things into your life if you don't believe you deserve them. I developed these three nets to support you in knowing that as an expression of Divine Light on Earth you deserve all things which are in your highest good.

The Sun Net

The Sun net is energising and masculine, or yang, in its action. Use it when there is a lack of confidence in personal power to achieve chosen goals, or a lack of motivation.

You will need: a golden yellow cloth, six rubies (small pinkish ones are affordable).

Lay the cloth out and space the crystals evenly to make a circle around yourself creating a six pointed Star of David. This layout may be done around you sitting up if space is limited. The outermost stones to each side should be within reach of your outstretched hands (relax your arms back to your sides when you've checked the circumference!)

Sit or lie in the net for up to 20 minutes whenever there is a need for self empowerment. Imagine the Sun is beaming upon you, warming you right through and filling your cell tissue with golden sunshine.

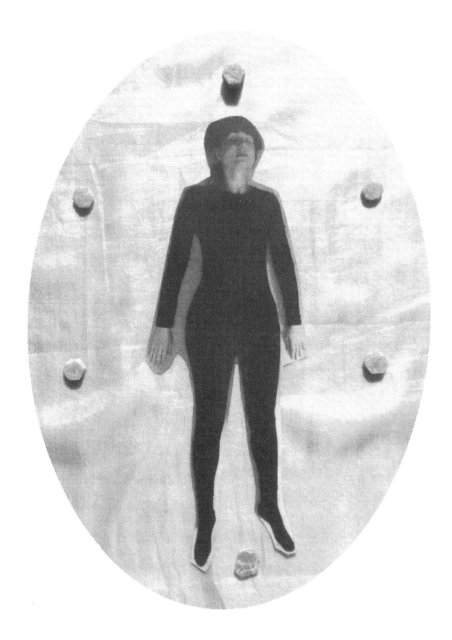

The Moon Net

The Moon Net is relaxing and feminine, or yin, in its action. Use it when you need to tap into your intuitive side and when you need to be receptive enough to welcome good things into your life.

You will need: a deep blue cloth, five moonstones

Lay the cloth out. Lie with arms and legs relaxed and open to create the star shape; you need to be open to receive. Place one stone above your head, one beneath the sole of each foot and hold one in each hand creating a five pointed star, or pentagram.

Lie in the net for up to 20 minutes whenever you feel a lack of deservingness, or that you are blocking the flow of energy in your life. Imagine Moonlight shining upon you and feel the cool radiance sweeping through you, cleansing and blessing you.

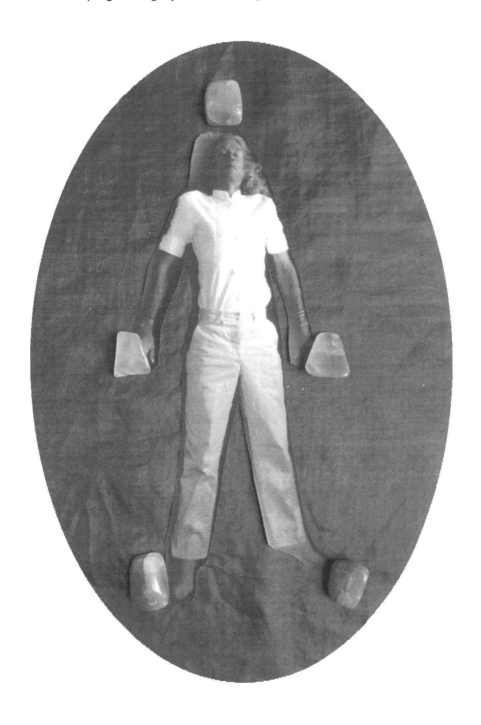

The Star Net

The Star Net takes you into contact with transpersonal energy. It is helpful for observing your actions from a higher viewpoint. Sometimes when things aren't turning out the way we hoped they would we need a less personal perspective, a more enlightened overview of what is going on. The Star Net reminds us that we are part of the magnificent web of the Universe and we are connected to all things. The seven clear stones invoke the energy of the Pleiades, or Seven Sisters. The cloth is black, mirroring the backdrop of the Universe and the Void from which all things come. Without the blackness we would not see the stars.

You will need: a black cloth, seven sparkling clear stones, small double terminated quartz such as Herkimer diamonds are ideal.

Lay the cloth out. Place the stones pointing inwards if they have single terminations. Place one stone above your head and one beneath each foot. Now place one stone on either side of your shoulders and one stone on either side of your hips, so that the stones create a seven pointed star, or elven star.

Lie in this net for up to 20 minutes and imagine you are being bathed in twinkling starlight. Know that you are making your contribution to the song of the Universe. You may find you perceive a higher viewpoint on your creations thus far and guidance on how to uplift your manifestations to a higher level.

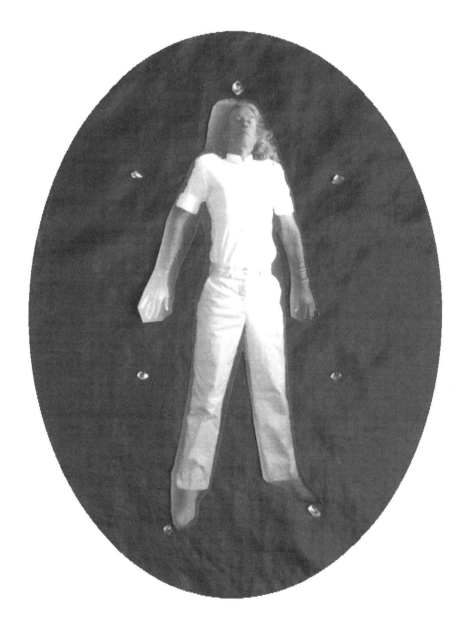

Chapter Ten:
Healing from a Far Eastern Perspective

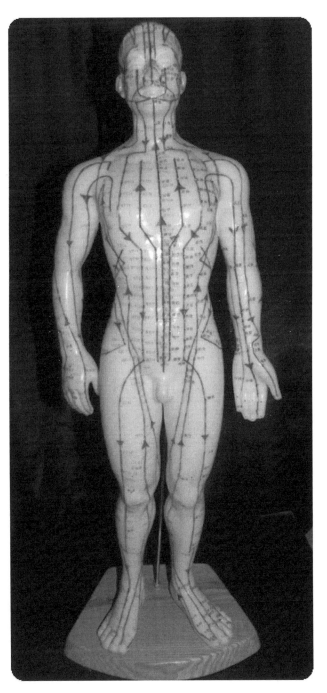

Yin and Yang

The well known yin yang symbol depicts the foundation of Traditional Chinese Medicine. It is a representation of the way that everything in the Universe is in a state of flux. Nothing remains the same, everything is always becoming either more yin or more yang.

Yin and yang can be understood most simply by looking at opposites:

Yin	Yang
female	male
passive	active
empty	full
dark	light
receiving	giving
winter	summer
night	day
soft	hard
black	white
cold	warm

When you look at the symbol the white yang swirl contains a dot of black yin energy at its fullest point and the black yin swirl contains a dot of white yang. Neither side dominates; it is a symbol of perfect balance and dynamic movement combined.

Everything can be compared against everything else as being more or less yin or yang and can be seen as moving towards one state or the other. Yin and yang is a relative concept:

To the frogs in a temple pool
The Lotus stems are tall;
To the gods of Mount Everest
An elephant is small.

Taoist Poem

For example Midsummer Solstice is the most yang time of the year, as it is the longest day, after which point the days become progressively more yin again. Autumn is more yin than Summer, but still has more yang energy than Winter. There are many natural cycles of change within us and the environment. Nothing is permanent and static. In understanding this we can accept the natural flow of change in our own lives more easily.

The quality of yin energy applied to human behaviour is stillness, quietude, restfulness, introversion, and solitude. The quality of yang is movement, noise, action, extroversion and sociability.

To live at either extreme is to be out of balance. Too much yin can lead to stagnation, apathy and depression, too much yang to depletion, anger, burn out and exhaustion.

When we are healthy we naturally move from one state to the other. After a hard day at work, being alert and busy, a yang state, our energy levels tend to drop and we need to relax. By spending a restful evening and having a good night's sleep, quiet yin time, we feel energetic and ready for action next day.

We need to acknowledge the action of yin and yang in our lives and go with the flow. Fighting life's natural fluctuations between busy and quiet, productive and fallow, sociability and solitude can lead to poor health. Make the most of the active times and enjoy resting and recuperating in the quiet ones, knowing that the tide will turn and bring busy times back to you once more and you will be refreshed and ready to participate again.

Most lifestyles tend to fall into 'more yin' or 'more yang' patterns and some people do get very out of balance and stuck in extremely yin or yang states. If there is too much yin the physical body may have illness caused by excess 'dampness', for example swollen limbs or excess mucous. An excess of yin may be expressed as tiredness and depression. A deficit of yin will result in dryness which can be seen in the skin and hair. Night sweats and other symptoms of the menopause may also be related to depleted yin.

If there is excess yang the skin tone may be reddish, there may be excessive activity, restlessness and issues with anger. Depleted yang shows as fatigue and poor concentration, if yang really becomes depleted there may be physical and mental exhaustion.

Apply the understanding of yin and yang to describe simple, common sense, practical ways to restore balance. For example if someone has a sedentary desk based job (yin) they'll need to take some exercise (yang), such as going for a walk at lunchtime. As with all crystal healing we intend to bring harmony and balance to the system.

Most crystals will have a 'more yin' or 'more yang' bias to their energy. Use more yang crystals in a healing on someone who is excessively yin to get their energy moving and more yin crystals on someone excessively yang to calm them and slow racing energy. You may need to choose stones less polarised than the examples below as very yang people can fight against relaxation and very yin people may need more gentle stimulation at first to get their energy going. Crystals with a Yin Yang balance are good general healing stones.

As a rule of thumb crystals with colours belonging to the warm end of the colour spectrum, the reds, oranges and yellows, will be more yang in action, whereas crystals which have colours belonging to the cool end of the spectrum, the blues, indigos and violets will be more yin in action. Green crystals tend to have a balance of yin yang energy.

Touchstones
Yin stones

Moonstone: enhances connection with the feminine, intuitive side of yourself.
Lepidolite: encourages acceptance of what is, peaceful and sedative.
Mangano calcite: soothes and nurtures, gives a gentle pink hug.
Selenite: clears stagnant energies, has a cooling action.
Blue lace agate: soothes, peaceful energy supports calm communication
Larimar: cools, refreshes, encourages heated emotions to settle.

Touchstones
Yang Stones

Sunstone: empowers and motivates into action, a fiery energy.
Red jasper: helps you stand your ground when necessary, assertive energy.
Iron pyrite: energises and supports an intention to move forward.
Citrine: supports a positive and optimistic outlook.
Carnelian: instils the confidence and courage to take action.
Ruby: stimulates life force energy and boosts enthusiasm.

Touchstones
Yin Yang Balance Stones

Emerald: promotes an even-handed, fair approach to others.
Super seven: grounds and uplifts, helps one remain centred.
Jade: balances action with wisdom, a stone of moderation.
Dalmatian jasper: uplifting whilst helping one to remain calm and peaceful.
Preseli bluestone: grounding whilst energising and empowering.
Lapis lazuli: this deep blue stone encourages introspection whilst the golden pyrite flecks assist communication of the wisdom gained by going within.

Chinese Five Element Theory

Five element theory considers that everything in the Universe is made up of the Chinese five elements: Fire, Earth, Metal, Water, Wood. It is interesting that in the West we have an ancient belief that everything is also made of five elements: Earth, Air, Fire, Water and Ether and there are some similarities between the two systems.

The Chinese Five Elements are not static, they are in a dynamic dance with each other and create the cycle of change. The relationship between the five elements is governed by the supportive and destructive cycle, as seen on the diagram below✓.

In the supportive cycle chi moves smoothly, each element supporting the next. However this supportive process is draining so each element is drained by the following one in the cycle. For example a tree is nourished by water, but in the process the water is used up. Similarly a fire is fed by wood, but in the process the wood is burned. In the destructive process the elements damage each other as the quote below describes:

"With Metal, wood is felled. With water, fire is extinguished. With wood, earth is rooted and loosened. With fire, metal is melted. And with earth, water is obstructed." Huang Di Nei Jing

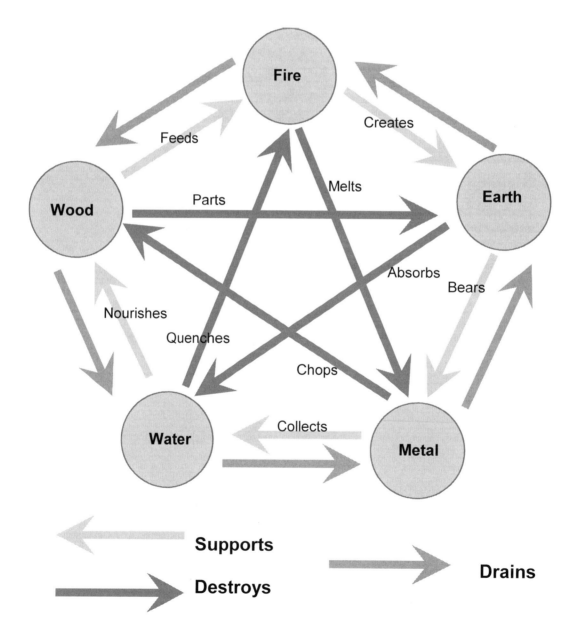

Feng Shui and Crystals

Feng Shui is an ancient Chinese system that aims to balance and harmonise energy as it circulates through a given space such as a home or workplace. In Feng Shui each direction is governed by one of the elements and has certain attributes as shown in the Lo Shu Square below.

Prosperity, Blessings and Abundance **South East** Main Cure: Wood Supported by: Water Destroyed by: Metal	Fame and Self expression **South** Main Cure: Fire Supported by: Wood Destroyed by: Water	Relationships and Marriage **South West** Main Cure: Earth Supported by: Fire Destroyed by: Wood
Family, Elders and Ancestors **East** Main Cure: Wood Supported by: Water Destroyed by: Metal	Unity and Health **Centre** Keep the centre clear. ensure energy circulates easily and is not blocked or drained here.	Children and Creativity **West** Main Cure: Metal Supported by: Earth Destroyed by: Fire
Education and Knowledge **North East** Main Cure: Earth Supported by: Fire Destroyed by: Wood	Career and Life Path **North** Main Cure: Water Supported by: Metal Destroyed by: Earth	Helpful Friends and Guides **North West** Main Cure: Metal Supported by: Earth Destroyed by: Fire

The Lo Shu square can be expanded and contracted to overlay any property or room and needs to be aligned to the compass points. To enhance the corresponding area of your life you should add objects, or 'cures' representing that element, or the supporting element for that area. Avoid having elements that drain or destroy the governing element in that area.

The Lo Shu square shows which directions which will be enhanced by the placement of crystals, which are a traditional Earth element cure. The North should be free of crystals.

In an ideal situation you would do your crystal therapy and store your crystals in one of the areas that respond well to Earth. My own healing room is in the North East of my home. If that isn't possible you can shrink the Lo Shu to cover the room you are using and enhance the appropriate areas of that room, so display your crystals in the South West or North East for example.

Typical Feng Shui Cures
Wood: houseplants, wooden furniture and objects, pictures of woodland
Fire: fireplace, lighting, candles
Earth: crystals and rocks, pottery
Metal: metallic objects, electronic equipment
Water: aquarium, indoor fountain, glassware, picture of natural water

NB. Feng Shui is a complete study in its own right and the information is offered here for the contemplation and assessment of your own living and therapy space, in particular your placement of crystals.

The Chinese Five Elements and the Five Phases of Change

There are five phases of change, each corresponding to one of the five elements. This is based on an observation that everything in nature goes through a natural cycle, the beginning, the expansion, the high point, stability, the retreat and the end.

Water = the beginning
Wood = the expansion
Fire = the high point
Earth = stability
Metal = the retreat
Water = the end

Notice the phase of Water is both at the beginning and the end which shows us that all of Nature is cyclical, in every ending there is a new beginning. Earth is the balance point. It is potentially an enduring state and in the right conditions that state can last a very long time, but everything in the material world comes to an end eventually. As Eckhart Tolle said, "Even the Sun will die."

We can observe the cycle of change in our human life cycle. We are born, grow as children, reach our full height potential as teenagers, mature into adulthood and then become middle aged, finally reaching old age and death. If you believe in reincarnation there is a rebirth and the cycle continues. Of course some people are 'middle aged' by the time they get to 40 and some remain youthful until they are past 60, whereas some are decidedly elderly by then. There is no fixed age where we transition between each phase.

The phases can apply to anything, whether it is a relationship, a job, a house or a body. When you are working on your own development, or working with a client, you can consider which of the phases of change applies. So if you have an exciting new project under development then it is likely to be in the Wood phase, where putting energy in will reap rapid growth and expansion. On the other hand if a job is losing its lustre it may be in Metal phase and perhaps looking for a fresh angle, taking on a new responsibility, or seeking a new job may need to be considered. Fighting the natural flow is not helpful. Everything has its time. Our lives are constantly evolving and old, spent aspects need to be released to allow fresh new growth to emerge.

Wood Element

The energy of Wood is new yang, the energy of new growth. It is the start of the day, the rising Sun in the East and it also governs the South East. It is the fresh shoots of Springtime, the unfurling leaves. The colour for Wood element is green.

Wood element corresponds to childhood and the rapid development of mind and body we experience at this time. Engage with Wood energy when you want to start new projects.

Touchstones

Tree agate: supports of new growth and development.
Aventurine: promotes fresh energy and inspiration for new ventures.
Serpentine: helps one to welcome change and supports your personal evolution.

Fire Element

The energy of Fire element is full yang, the culmination, or the high point of any situation. It is midday, when the Sun is at its zenith. It corresponds to direction of the South, to warmth and Summer. The colour of Fire element is red.

In human terms it corresponds to our teenage years when we reach our height potential and are at our most excitable. Utilise Fire element when you need more joie de vivre or get up and go, or when you just need warmth, either physically or emotionally.

> **Touchstones**
> **Ruby:** stimulates a passionate engagement with life and promotes vitality.
> **Sunstone:** supports joie de vivre and a zest for living.
> **Rhodonite:** encourages one to share personal talents and strengths.

Earth Element

Sitting in the middle of the cycle of change Earth element exhibits a balance of yin and yang. Earth is solid and dependable, the most stable of the elements. It is the energy of afternoon and late Summer. It governs the South West and North East. The colour for Earth is yellow or brown.

In human terms Earth corresponds to adulthood. Depending on our lifestyle and constitution the Earth phase of our lives can span many decades. If you need security and stability in your life utilise Earth element.

> **Touchstones**
> **Amber:** warms and soothes at the same time, nurtures and harmonises.
> **Mookaite:** steadies, encourages down to earth practicality.
> **Tiger's eye:** promotes dynamic groundedness and a well-balanced outlook on life.

Metal Element

Metal is the energy of new yin and contraction, or accumulation. It is the evening and it governs the directions of West and North West. This is the energy of Autumn, when Nature bears fruit.

In human terms it is middle age when hopefully the hard work and energy you have put in is allowing you to reap returns. Turn to Metal when you have put the effort in and are ready to receive the rewards.

> **Touchstones**
> **Amethyst:** purifies and cleanses on all levels, brings peace and calm.
> **Rutilated quartz:** encourages connection, promotes recuperation and repair.
> **Iron Pyrites:** the golden colour represents the energy of abundance and prosperity.

Water Element

Water is the energy of full yin and of conservation or retreat. It is the night and governs the direction of North. This is the energy of Winter, the quietest, stillest time of the year when much lays hidden.

In human terms it corresponds to old age. You have done your work and now it is time to rest and simply be. Call on Water when you need to retreat from the hustle and bustle of the world for a while.

> **Touchstones**
> **Aquamarine:** encourages one to be still and replenish reserves.
> **Blue apatite:** cleanses, facilitates the release of old emotional patterns.
> **Kyanite:** offers detachment from situations where your energy is enmeshed.

The Meridians

The meridians are subtle energy channels carrying chi energy. At first glance there appears to be no correlation between the meridians shown on the charts and the organ names they are given. This is because only the sections of the channels which run close to the surface of the skin are shown on most acupuncture charts. These are the accessible channels which may be treated with acupuncture needles, or in our case with crystals. In actual fact the meridians also run deeper into the body and connect with their given organs, but as these channels are too deep to access with needles they are not shown on most charts. If you are interested in further study Sue Hix's Fourteen Classical Meridians shows these deeper channels as dotted lines.

Twelve of the meridians are pairs running on the left and right side of the body as mirror images of each other. Two additional meridians run on the midline of the body, front and back. Each meridian has a series of points located upon it. The points are places where the energy of the meridian may be accessed and are where acupuncture needles would be used. On some charts you will see that the points are individually numbered. The points have traditional names and specific attributes which an acupuncturist would study.

Acupuncturists must develop a precise awareness of where the acupuncture points are as they will be inserting fine needles to stimulate the energy. We are fortunate as we will be applying crystals which are non-invasive and have a much larger surface area, plus their own energy field surrounding them. We can afford to be 'close enough', although the more accurately you can locate the points the better.

Acupuncture points often feel tender when pressed gently. You need to familiarise yourself with the feel of them before working on others. As you look through the following charts I suggest you select a meridian to trace on your own body, preferably one that you feel you may have an issue with. On the charts I have added an arrow to indicate flow. It is important to note this as you should work in the direction of the flow of chi to strengthen the meridian. Begin at the start point and at each point location press gently for a moment and notice how it feels. Do this with both the left and right side. Do not do this with more than one meridian at a time or you are likely to precipitate a healing crisis for yourself!

I added the black lines and arrows to my mannequin as they help me check the position and flow of each meridian. Mannequins are readily available from stores selling equipment for acupuncture and are useful as you can see the meridians from every angle.

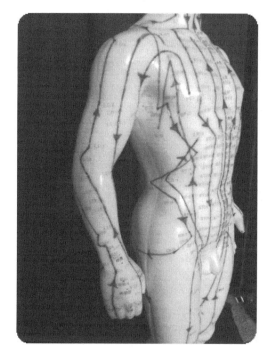

The Organ Clock

The Organ Clock shows the progression of energy through the meridians over 24 hours. Each meridian has high and low phases through the day. The lowest phase is 12 hours after the peak time. You can use the clock to identify which meridian is most in need of treatment. If there is a regular time when symptoms show up, worsen, or vitality levels slump, or if there are regular times of waking in the night then you need to consider whether it is the meridian that is at its highest phase or the one at its lowest ebb. Excessive functioning will usually manifest disturbance during the peak time of that meridian's function, suppressed function may manifest at the lowest time. Look at the description given for each meridian and see whether there is a match for the symptoms being experienced.

You can work on meridians at any time of day, however the organ clock shows us the most effective times and this is useful advice to pass onto clients for self treatment at home. The six hours before the peak time are when the energy is rising and so these are also beneficial times to treat. We do have to be practical. It is best to self treat the meridians that are active in the night just before bedtime. A client can be shown how to self treat at home and given an appropriate stone to work with.

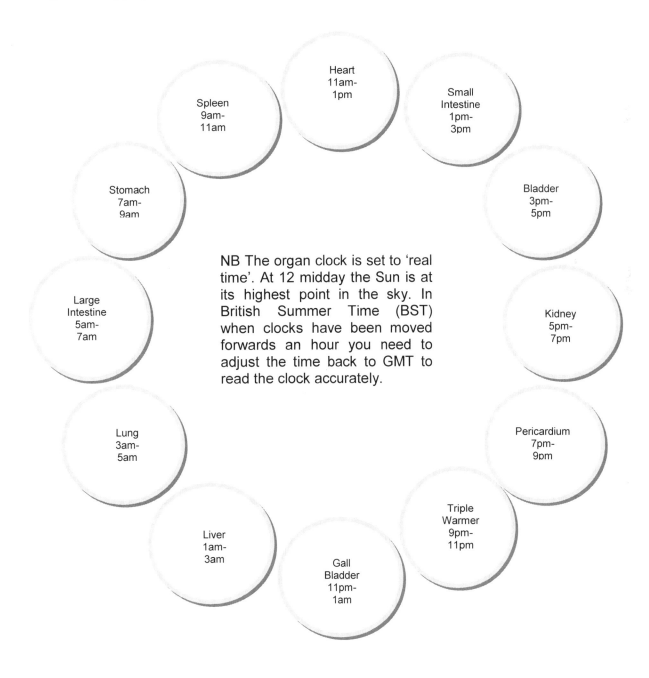

NB The organ clock is set to 'real time'. At 12 midday the Sun is at its highest point in the sky. In British Summer Time (BST) when clocks have been moved forwards an hour you need to adjust the time back to GMT to read the clock accurately.

Traditional Chinese Medicine recommends 'best times' to do things based on the meridian clock. These may not fit in with Western lifestyles, however the closer we follow the guidance the more we work with, rather than against, our natural flow of energy. It doesn't mean you only do that thing at that time, just that these are the optimum two hours of the day to do the recommended activity. You are not expected to spend two hours eating your breakfast! You can also extrapolate 'worst times' for activities which are 12 hours later when the associated meridian energy is at its lowest ebb.

5am-7am:	Bowel Movement
7am-9am:	Breakfast
9am-11am:	Digestion
11am-1pm:	Stay Calm
1pm-3pm:	Eat Lunch
3pm-5pm:	Have meetings
5pm-7pm:	Wind Down
7pm-9pm:	Supper & romance
9pm-11pm:	Warmth & Lovemaking
11pm-1am:	Clear the Mind
1am-3am:	Calm the emotions
3am-5am:	Meditation

If you prefer a more intuitive approach to working on the meridians you can use the dowsing chart opposite to choose which meridian is the priority for treatment.

Meridian Dowsing Chart

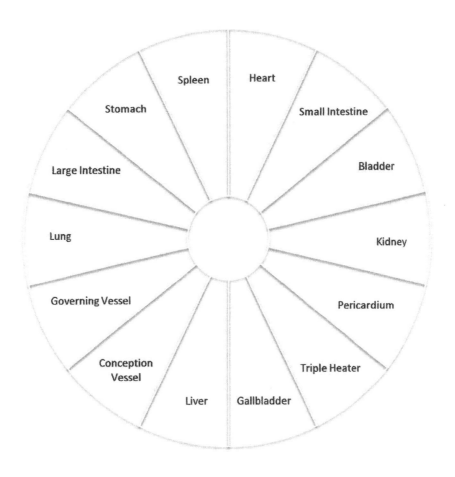

Lung Meridian

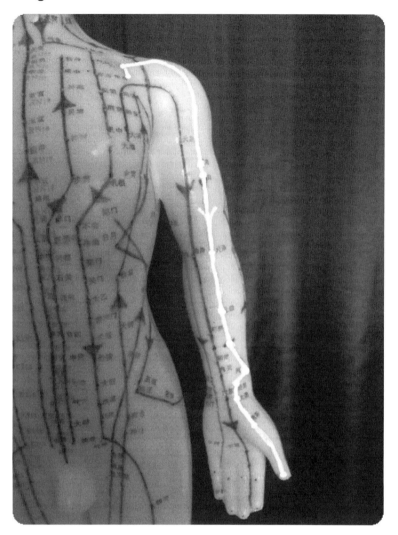

Yin

Metal Element

3am-5am GMT   4am-6am BST

Start Point: At shoulder between first and second ribs.
End Point: Thumb

Signs of Dysfunction:
Either shunning physical closeness or overstepping boundaries to get inappropriately close.
Respiratory illnesses including persistent coughs, asthma and bronchitis.

Self Help Tips:
Indulge in physical affection, whether that is with loved ones or pets.
Have a massage.
Do breathing exercises.
Do exercise that works with the breath such as yoga or Tai Chi.
Avoid substances that harm the lungs such as cigarette smoke, dusty environments and solvents.

Large Intestine Meridian

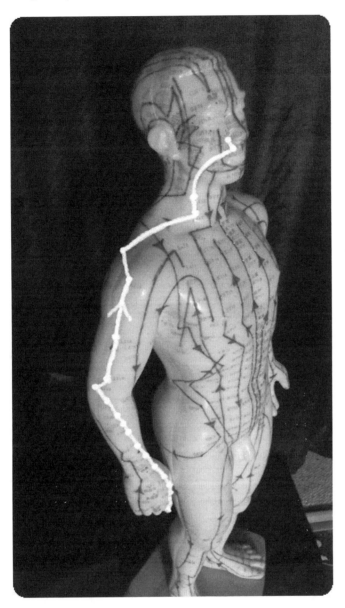

Yang

Metal Element

5am-7am GMT   6am-8am BST

Start Point: Index finger
End Point: Beside nostril

Signs of Dysfuntion:
Issues with letting go and stubborness, or inability to hold onto things.
Constipation or diarrhea.

Self Help Tips:
Wash in the morning whilst consciously letting go of accumulated heavy energies.
Clear out clutter and junk, especially let go of possessions which remind you of sad or difficult times.

Stomach Meridian

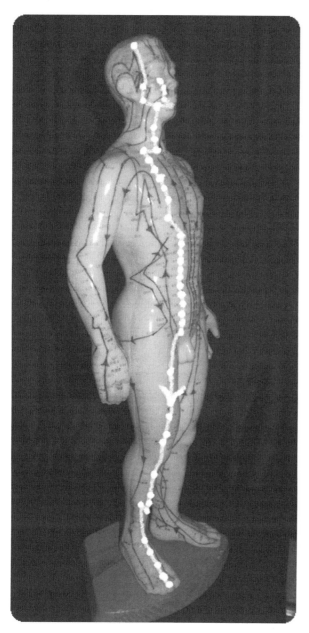

Yang

Earth Element

7am-9am GMT   8am-10am BST

Start point: Under eye
End Point: Second toe

Signs of Dysfunction:
Inability to discern between what is good for wellbeing and what is not.
Digestive disorders including heartburn and indigestion, cravings and addictions.

Self Help Tips:
Eat well balanced nutritious meals, including breakfast and chew food properly.
Conduct a life review noting what is working well and what is holding you back.

Spleen Meridian

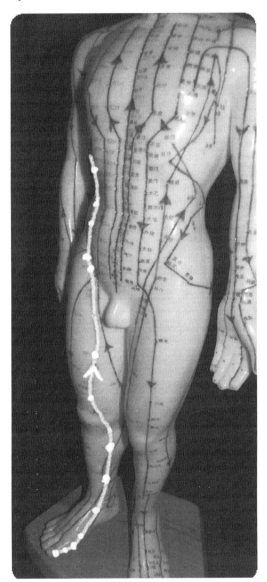 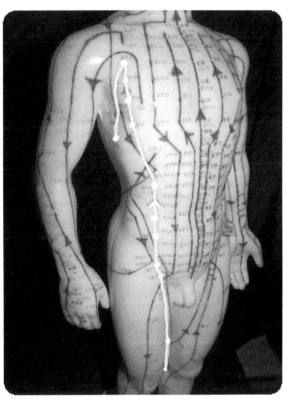

Yin

Earth Element

9am-11am GMT   10am-12 midday BST

Start Point: Big toe
End point: Below armpit

Signs of Dysfunction:
Poor stamina and lack of ability to plan and follow through, criticism of self or others.
Dietary deficiencies caused by inabilty to extract nutrients efficiently.

Self Help Tips:
Create a secure space as a safe base from which you move out into the world.
Find a system of planning that works for you and stick with it.

Heart Meridian

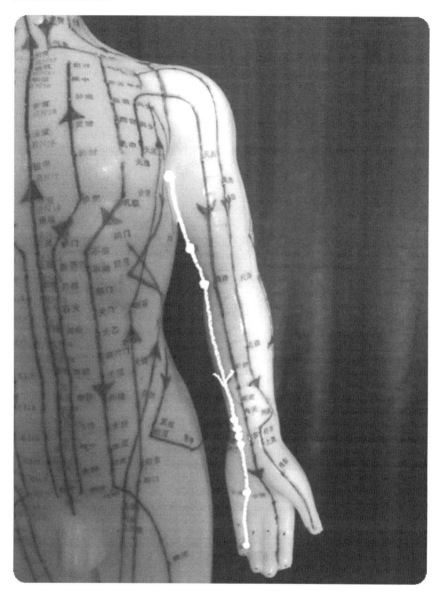

Yin

Fire Element

11am-1pm GMT   12 midday-2pm BST

Start Point: Armpit
End point: Little finger

Signs of Dysfunction:
Lack of empathy, hard heartedness, or oversensitive and pitying.
Insomnia, palpitations, stress.

Self Help Tips:
Build time for rest and relaxation into each day.
Create the conditions for a good night's sleep; dark room, comfortable pillows etc.

Small Intestine Meridian

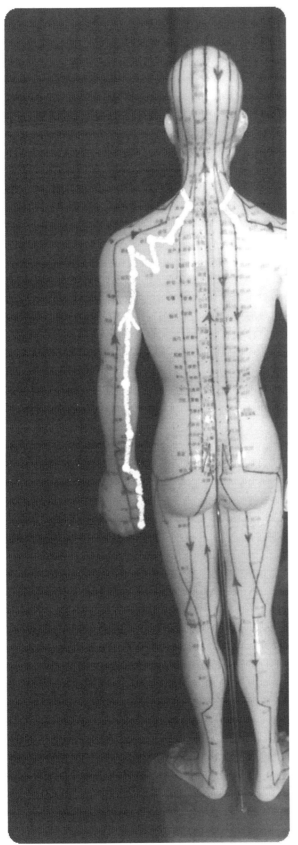

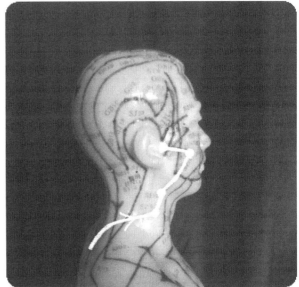

Yang

Fire Element

1pm-3pm GMT   2pm-4pm BST

Start point: Little finger
End point: By ear

Signs of Dysfunction:
Inability to discern between what is helpful and what is a hindrance.
Over involvement in other people's affairs, or lack of interest beyond the self.

Self Help Tips:
Take a rest after each meal to allow for proper assimilation of food.
Stand back from other people's lives and ask what motivates your involvement.

Bladder Meridian

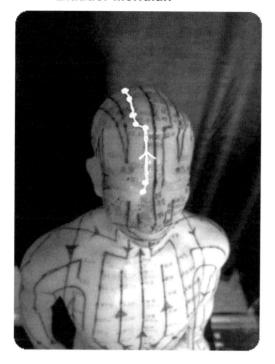

Yang

Water Element

3pm-5pm GMT   4pm-6pm BST

Start point: By eye
End point: Little toe

Signs of Dysfunction:
Over controlling behaviour, or
feeling a lack of control in your
life. Urinary disorders

Self Help Tips:
Drink water.
Swim, or spend time by water in
Nature.

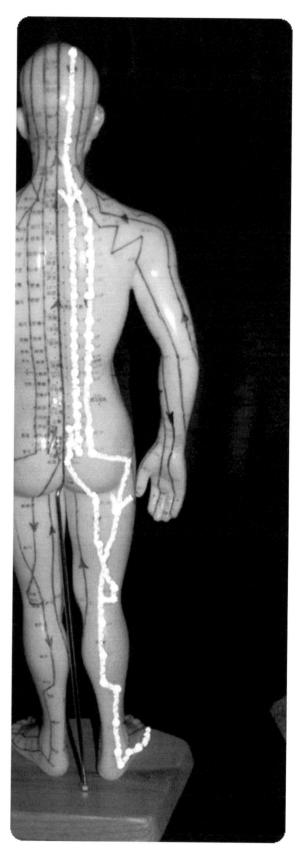

Kidney Meridian

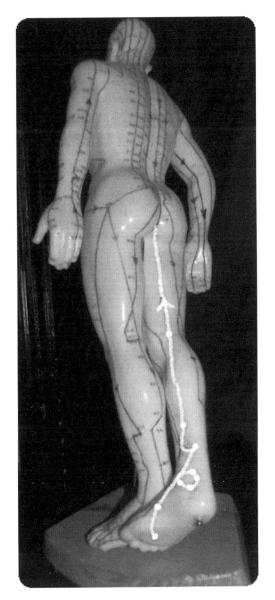
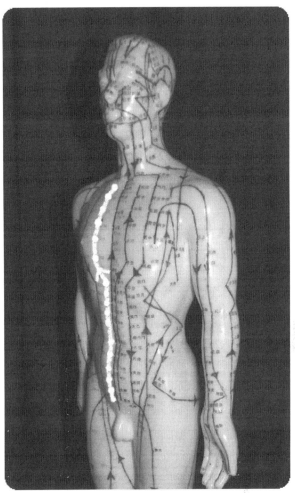

Yin

Water Element

5pm-7pm GMT   6pm-8pm BST

Start point: Sole of foot
End point: Under clavicle

Signs of Dysfunction:
Domineering behaviour or weakness of will.
Lack of vitality.

Self Help Tips:
Drink water.
Swim or spend time by water in Nature.

Pericardium / Heart Protector Meridian

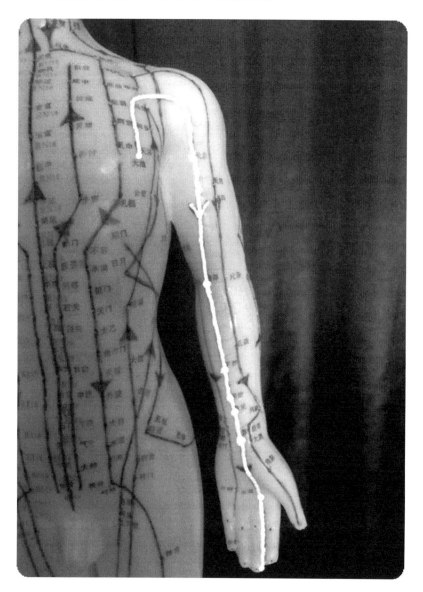

Yin

Fire Element

7pm-9pm GMT   8pm-10pm BST

Start Point: By nipple
End Point: Middle finger

Signs of Dysfunction:
Inability to relax and enjoy life and its physical pleasures.
Anxiety, nervousness.

Self Help Tips:
Take time out for relaxation.
Enjoy being in your sensual body, dance or enjoy intimacy.

Triple Heater Meridian

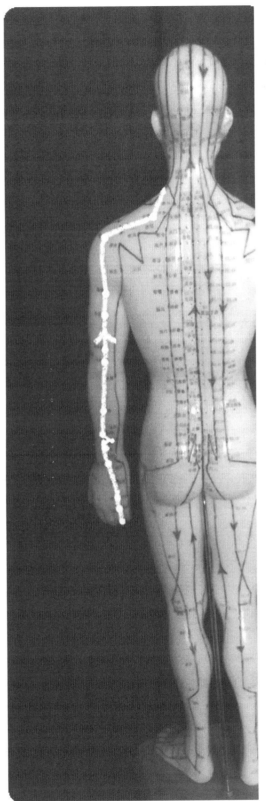

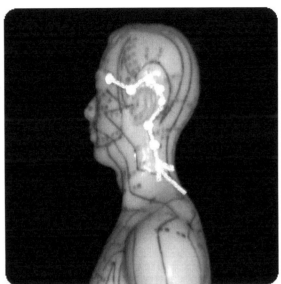

Yang

Fire Element

9pm-11pm GMT   10pm-12 midnight BST

Start Point: Ring finger
End Point: By eyebrow

Signs of Dysfunction:
Emotions either locked down, or gushing.
Distribution of body heat poorly
controlled, either feeling too hot or too
cold.

Self Help Tips:
Wear seasonal clothing, wear layers if
you veer between too hot and too cold.
Eat temperature appropriate foods,
cooling in summer, warming in winter.

Gall Bladder Meridian

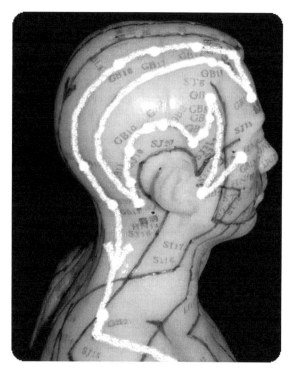

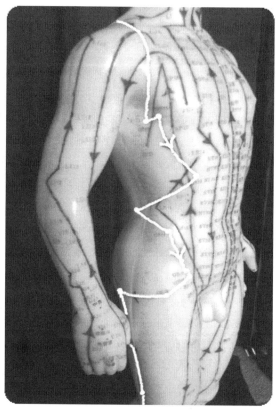

Yang

Wood Element

11pm-1am GMT 12 midnight-2am BST

Start Point: By eye
End Point: Fourth toe

Signs of Dysfunction:
Feeling trapped and making knee-jerk
decisions, or prevaricating and
procrastinating.
Headaches and migraines.

Self Help Tips
Be in bed resting by 11pm in the winter or
by midnight BST.
Pause and do deep breathing exercises
before trying to make any difficult
decisions.

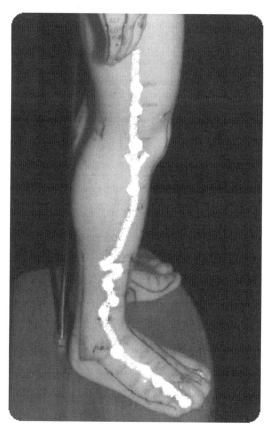

Liver Meridian

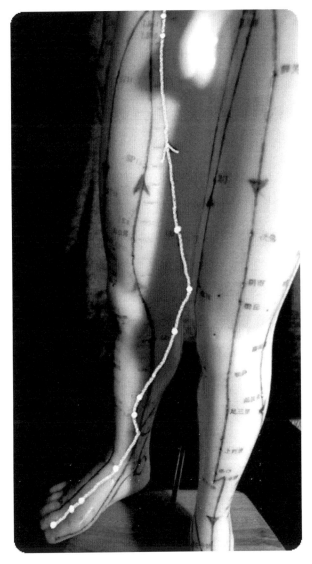 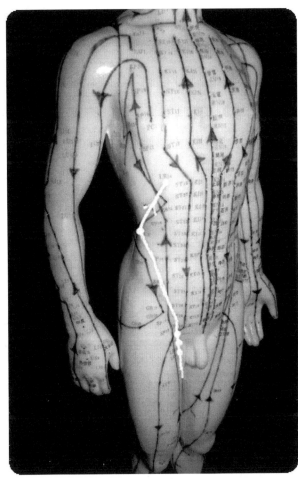

Yin

Wood Element

1am-3am GMT   2am-4am BST

Start Point: Big toe
End Point: On ribcage

Signs of Dysfunction:
Suppressed emotions and angry outbursts, or inability to move forwards with plans.
Stiffness in body and rigidly held points of view.

Self Help Tips:
Release blocked emotions by shouting where no-one can hear, or having a good cry.
Do exercise to promote flexibility such as yoga, walk in woods, try seeing the other side of an argument.

The Conception Vessel

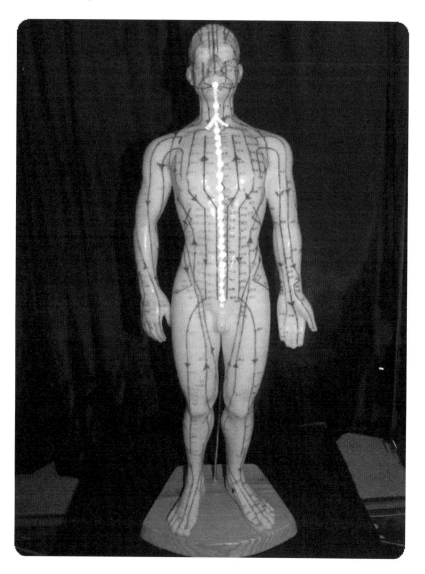

Connects all Yin Meridians internally.

No specific element.
No specific time.

Start Point: Perineum
End Point: Beneath lower lip

Signs of Dysfunction:
Issues with more than one of the Yin meridians would indicate a need to check the
Conception Vessel.

Yin Meridians:
Lung
Spleen
Heart
Kidney
Pericardium
Liver

The Governing Vessel

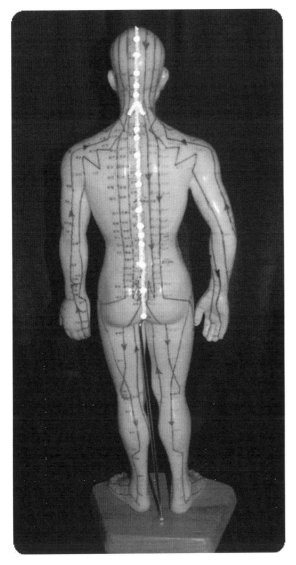
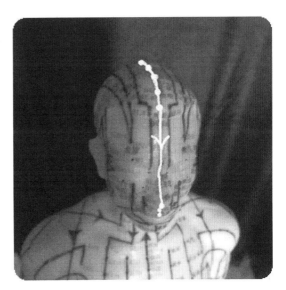

Connects all Yang meridians internally.

No specific element.
No specific time.

Start Point: Perineum
End Point: Upper lip

Signs of Dysfunction:
Issues with more than one of the Yang meridians
would indicate a need to check the Governing Vessel.

Yang Meridians:
Large Intestine
Stomach
Small Intestine
Bladder
Triple Heater
Gall Bladder

Treatment of Meridians

Treatment of Meridian End Points

- Prepare yourself for healing as usual.
- Locate which meridian to work with by dowsing, using the organ clock, or by considering symptoms.
- Turn to the diagram of that meridian.
- Intuit or dowse whether you need to work on the left or right side of the body first.
- Check whether a crystal needs to be used at either the start or end point.
- Choose a crystal appropriate for the Chinese element of that meridian.
- Dowse or intuit how long the crystal needs to be left in place and either hold the crystal in position or tape it as appropriate.
- When completed remove the crystal.
- If you treated the start point check whether you also need to treat the end point and repeat the procedure if so. Use a fresh crystal each time, or cleanse the one you have used.
- Dowse or intuit whether the same meridian on the other side of the body also needs a treatment in which case repeat the procedure.

Treatment of Specific Acupuncture Points

- Prepare yourself for healing as usual.
- Locate which meridian to work with by dowsing, using the organ clock, or by considering symptoms.
- Turn to the diagram of that meridian.
- Determine whether you need to work on the left or right side of the body first.
- Find the specific acupuncture point by dowsing along the meridian chart in the direction of the flow of energy.
- Choose a crystal appropriate for the Chinese element of the meridian.
- Locate the corresponding point on your client. Your client can help by applying *gentle* pressure around that area. Acupuncture points often feel tender. As you become more sensitive you may sense the subtle energy of these points.
- Dowse or intuit how long the crystal needs to be left in place and either hold the crystal in position or tape it as appropriate.
- When completed remove the crystal.
- Check whether any further points along that meridian need treatment by dowsing the diagram in the direction of the flow. Repeat the procedure until you have ascertained that no further points on that meridian need any treatment. Use a fresh crystal each time, or cleanse the one you have used.
- When the treatment on that meridian is completed check whether the same meridian on the other side of the body also needs treatment and repeat the procedure if so.

Important Note

Like water meridian energy will flow along the path of least resistance. If you are holding a crystal on your client at a place of blockage you may notice a tingling running up your hand and arm. This is energy leaking, using your own meridians as the path of least resistance. This is not helpful for your client.

Use your intention to stop this happening, or prevent this occurrence by using micropore tape rather than holding the crystal in place.

General Application

This is a simple method for self treatment and for clients to use between sessions. Remember to explain cleansing crystals to clients.

- Dowse which meridian needs ongoing support. This may be the one you have worked with in the therapy session, or it could be another, often the other meridian controlled by the same element, so for example you may have worked on the Bladder Meridian as the priority, but the Kidney Meridian may also need support.

- Dowse or intuit whether the left side, right side, or both sides of the Meridian need treatment.

- Suggest appropriate crystals for your client to work with.

- Looking at the Meridian charts see where the Meridian flows to ascertain whether the best results will be obtained by placing the crystal/s at the wrists, ankles or around the neck over the thymus.

- Dowse how often the stone needs to be applied and how long for.

- If the stone needs to be worn over a longer period of time it can be held in place by a elasticated wrist or ankle support bandage, as a pendant, or power bracelets can be put into therapeutic use.

A Note on Using Micropore Tape

Micropore tape is handy as it will hold stones in place so that you or your client don't have to. For any of these methods you may tape the stone in place. The tape can leave stones a bit sticky, so only use it with stones that you can wash in soapy water.

Check a client is happy with your use of micropore and do not use on any sensitive or delicate areas of the body. Avoid use on irritated or broken skin. Micropore can be stuck to clothing and usually leaves little residue behind, but it can pull threads on its removal so use your judgement and common sense; jeans are generally okay, designer mohair not a good idea for example! If in doubt hold the stone in place instead. You can purchase micropore tape easily from chemists and most supermarkets.

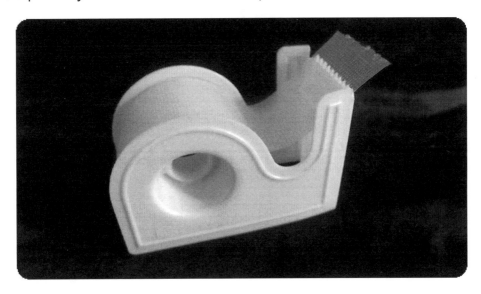

Chapter Eleven:
The Holistic Spine

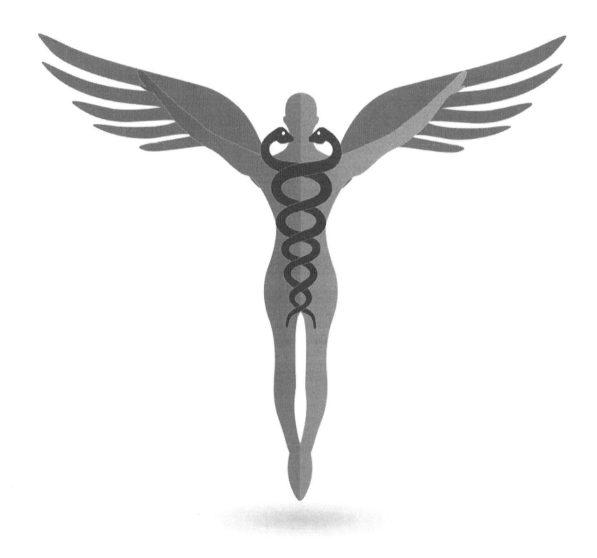

The Holistic Spine

The spine is the largest conduit of life force energy through the body. Clearing the energy in the spine can aid wellbeing on every level. In the Indian tradition the spine is depicted as having a central channel of prana termed the Sushumna which when clear allows the free flow of energy from Heaven to Earth and Earth to Heaven.

There are two other major currents that criss-cross at the chakra points starting at the base of the spine and ending at each nostril. These are called Ida and Pingala. Ida starts on the left side, ends at the left nostril and is a feminine current, aligned to lunar energy. Pingala starts on the right side and ends at the right nostril, is masculine and solar in nature. Clearing these two currents helps us achieve integration and balance between our receptive and active natures and helps to keep all the chakras functioning in a healthy way.

These energy channels are termed nadis, a Sanskrit word meaning 'streams'. There are many more nadis in the body, however these three are the largest channels.

It is interesting that the shape produced by the three main energy channels up the spine is the same as the Staff of Hermes, otherwise known as the Caduceus, which has long been used as a symbol for the medical profession and healing. This shows a largely unconscious recognition of the importance of these three currents which have been recognised in healing since ancient times.

The main chakras all feed into the central column of spinal energy. It is not uncommon to develop back problems where a chakra is blocked or functioning poorly, so a chakra balance can be beneficial. The Chinese meridian system also underlines the importance of the spine, with the Governing vessel running up the centre back of the body.

As back pain is a primary cause of time off work every year and can be debilitating, care for the energy of the spine is important on the physical level alone. Additionally our other physical systems are linked into the back, which is not surprising when you think of the role of the central nervous system in carrying messages to and from parts of the body.

We can store our emotional issues in our spine. Chiropractic diagrams of the spine can be illuminating. A bad back can tell a therapist a lot about what is going on for a client! I refer to a wall chart by John Cross Clinics which contains a wealth of information about physical ailments and emotional issues that arise from specific spinal misalignments.

The diagram on the following page can be used to help locate back issues and to keep written records of where you needed to apply crystals.

Kundalini Energy

Kundalini is a natural energy that everyone possesses. The Hindu tradition depicts the energy as the serpent Kundalini wound three and a half times around the base chakra. In most people she lies dormant at the base of the spine and stays sleeping throughout their lifetime. There are spiritual practices developed specifically to awaken Kundalini, such as Kundalini Yoga. These are adhered to because Kundalini holds primal power and raising the energy can lead to a blissful and enlightening connection with the Divine.

You should not try to awaken Kundalini energy for a client. Woken prematurely Kundalini can wreak merry havoc, shooting strong energy up the spine and causing great discomfort and pain wherever it runs into blocks. These may be at chakra points or elsewhere in the spine. Kundalini can cause diverse symptoms that are strong, even overwhelming, such as back pain and headaches, hot flushes, shaking and panicky feelings. Once awakened it seems futile to try to push Kundalini back down the spine. This is akin to trying to get the genie back in the bottle! The natural flow of Kundalini is up the spine and out through the crown chakra.

The most helpful way I've found to assist someone who is struggling with Kundalini symptoms is to clear the channel of the spine using the techniques in this chapter so that this powerful energy can rise smoothly without obstruction. Teach them to ground themselves as this is essential for staying secure through this experience and provides a natural way to discharge excessive energy building up in their system.

Cervical spinal segments
and roots

Thoracic spinal segments
and roots

Lumbal spinal segments
and roots

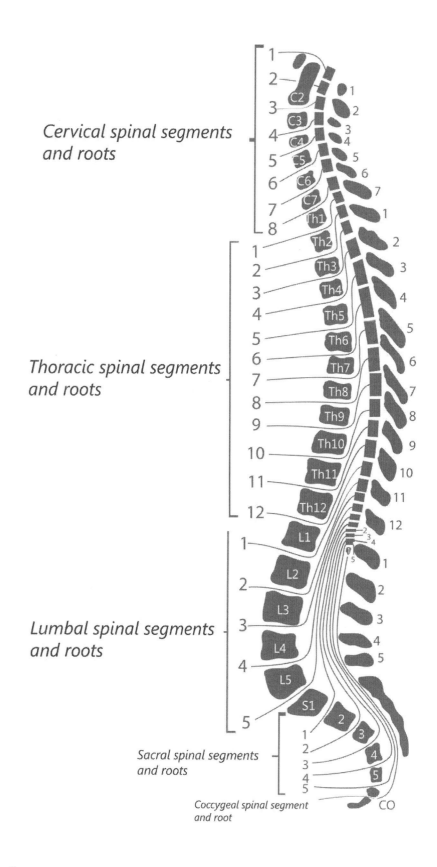

Sacral spinal segments
and roots

Coccygeal spinal segment
and root

Healing the Spine

One of the best ways to consciously clear the energy in the spine is through using the breath. A powerful exercise is to stand or sit upright and visualise breathing energy up your spine from the base chakra on the in breath and down your spine again on the out breath. Each time you breathe in you raise the energy a little further. You may find it will only rise to a certain level, indicating a blockage for you to work on releasing.

You may imagine that the rising breath flows out of your Crown and connects you with the Divine and that the descending breath flows into the ground connecting you to Mother Earth. If you are standing and feel light headed at any point sit down, focus on the contact your feet are making with the ground and go back to breathing normally. Always finish on the out breath as this leaves you feeling grounded. If you do this simple exercise for just a few minutes every morning you may be surprised by the difference in your overall vitality.

Yoga makes use of alternate nostril breathing to help clear and balance the Ida and Pingala nadis. By closing off one nostril and breathing in through the other you stimulate the associated nadi, so if at some point in your day you need more vitality and dynamism spend a couple of minutes breathing in through your right nostril and out through your left nostril. If you feel stressed and you need more inner peace and receptivity breathe in through your left nostril and out through your right nostril. For general practice allow time to work on both sides as you risk causing an imbalance by just focussing on one side.

Doing regular exercise that keeps the back supple, such as yoga, pilates or bellydance is helpful. Getting a back massage can release a lot of tension, and finding a good chiropractor is wise if you feel your back needs more physical manipulation. Crystal therapy can be used to complement physical therapies as we work on the flow of energy and they can correct physical alignment.

Awareness of your posture will help the energy flow well both when standing and sitting. Imagine a golden thread connects the crown of your head up to the heavens so that you are suspended from it. Allow the rest of your body to come into alignment and balance below. This is a quick, but effective way to check your posture and can make a real difference.

Crystal Healing for the Spine

Some people find lying face down very uncomfortable. If I am working on a client's spine I normally do that part of their treatment first so that they can turn over and relax for the rest of the session. If you have a couch with a face hole or a face cradle it is a bit more comfortable. The use of an amethyst cluster is suitable for someone who can't lie face down.

Using an Amethyst Cluster

With your client sitting on a stool, or sideways on a chair so their back is accessible, hold a hand sized amethyst cluster and work in the etheric body, approximately 2-3cm away from the physical body. Use rhythmic flowing strokes to work from the top of the head and down the centre line of the spine as if you are brushing long hair. Blockages will feel denser. You will sense the strokes becoming more smooth and easy as you clear the energy. Pause to cleanse the amethyst cluster if it starts to feel heavy.

A Chakra Balance on the Rear Chakras

Whilst crystal therapists normally do chakra balancing with the client lying on their back, you can ask your client to lie face down instead and place the crystals directly on the rear chakras. People with back pain often have blocked chakras in the area of the discomfort.

A 'One Line' Clearing

With your client lying face down you can adapt the five line clearing method using a pendulum with your focus on clearing the first line up the centre spine. You can of course go on to clear the other lines too if your client is comfortable enough and you sense it would be beneficial.

Using Double-terminated Quartz (DTs)

Double-terminated quartz crystals are especially effective on the spine as they help the energy flow in both directions, upwards and downwards. With your client lying face down use your pendulum to dowse along the spine to find where the DTs need placing. You are asking for the pendulum to show you any breaks, blockages or disruption in the flow of energy. Where the pendulum changes its spin place the DTs. If it is a long area or you only have small DTs you can arrange several crystals end to end as pictured.

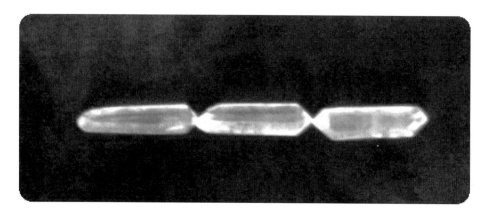

Once the problem area is identified and covered by the DT crystals you can then use your pendulum, a massage wand, or a milky quartz point to draw off any stagnated energy off from that area.

Once the area feels clearer you can re-energise it by directing energy through a clear quartz point. Finally smooth and seal over the area with selenite before removing the DTs.

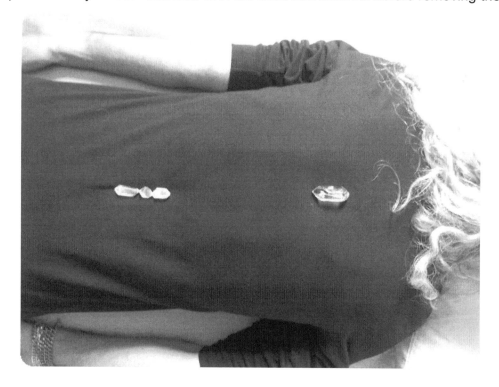

Chapter Twelve:
Distant Healing

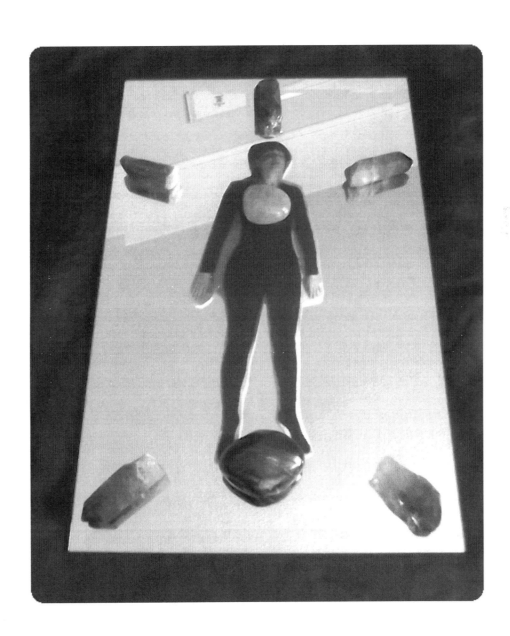

Distant Healing

Distant healing, also referred to as absent healing, is a way of sending or receiving healing energy when the client cannot be present with you. The obvious advantage is that it can reach people, places and animals anywhere in the world as energy has no boundaries and reaches its destination virtually instantaneously.

Healers, churches and other religious groups have been sending healing energy out into the world for a very long time, often in the form of prayer. When you are distant healing with crystals the crystal energy will find its recipient through the power of your intention.

When you are thinking of sending distant healing there are a few ethical issues to consider. The first is whether you have conscious permission from the intended recipient. Do they actually want the healing? Not everyone feels comfortable with the idea of receiving crystal healing. I feel that any adult who has the ability to make a choice has the right to be asked if this is something they want, otherwise it is an invasion of their privacy and an interference in their personal energy field. The tendency of some practitioners to send healing to anyone they can think of who is sick may be well intentioned but it is not respectful of other people's boundaries.

The exceptions to this rule are for children, where their parent or guardian can ask for the healing and for someone unable to ask for themselves, such as someone in a coma or with severe mental impairment. In these extreme circumstances next of kin may give permission on their behalf.

You do not have to meet your client in person before setting them up in distant healing. I have clients who live in America and in Europe. With communication possible via telephone, Skype, email or text you can keep yourself updated with a client's progress and work very effectively. Ensure you record what you have done in the same way that you would with your client present.

It is worth making the distinction between sending healing to a named individual and sending healing to an area or a group of people. Where people are suffering in the world, for example in war zones or through famine, then the sending of healing to those places is a positive action. Those who are open to receive the healing energy may benefit, yet it is not focussed upon any one individual.

Take energy safety seriously. Before you begin prepare your energy just as carefully as you would for a healing with the client present. It is easy to be blasé without the person in front of you, but as you tune in to set up the healing you are in effect making an energetic connection between yourself and the recipient. Remember to disconnect from your client once the healing is set up.

Obtaining a Witness

Request a photograph of the recipient. You can work with a head and shoulders image, but a full body (clothed!) image is useful. This photograph is known as a 'witness'. You may take a photograph at a client's appointment with their permission as this gives you a way to check and stabilise their energy from a distance if they report a healing crisis, or if they cannot visit you in person, but would still like a treatment. Store their photograph safely with their notes.

In days gone by locks of hair, nail clippings or blood were used as witnesses because these carry the unique DNA of the individual, however with the advent of digital cameras, email and mobile phones a photo is usually quick and easy to obtain. I find it helps greatly with the selection and layout of crystals if I can see the person I am working on. If you really want the DNA link then ask for a small lock of hair taped to a photo to be posted to you. Nail clippings and blood samples are best avoided for hygiene purposes. Alternatively an accurate astrological birth chart may appeal to those with a background in astrology. You could also use a sample of handwriting and a signature as a witness.

Using a Sending Device

A sending device is usually a shiny flat surface which will help to send the crystal energy off to the recipient. You can use a clean mirror tile, which are quite inexpensive and available in a useful range of sizes from DIY stores, or sometimes sold as 'candle plates'. Also effective, though harder to obtain, are polished crystal slabs, quartz being the most universal energy. Bear in mind that the crystals used as sending devices will make a difference to the healing. Pictured below are a polished rock quartz slab and a lepidolite book.

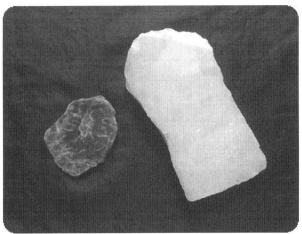

Copper is an excellent conductor of energy, so you could use a polished copper sheet. My husband Steve made me a couple of beautiful copper and crystal healing plates which are excellent to use. You could make a simple version with a sheet of copper, wire and some quartz points.

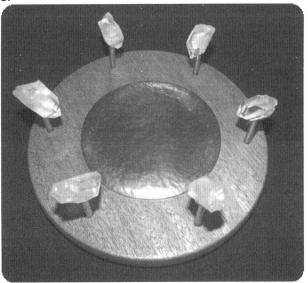

Using a Flat Based Polished Quartz Point

Nice quality quartz crystals are often polished and given a flat base so that they stand upright. I have found these are excellent placed on the distant healing to gather all of the crystal energies you have placed and send them as a coherent beam.

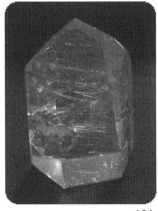

Sending Distant Healing with Crystals

- In preparation talk to the client about what they are hoping for from the healing and agree a day or time that you will be putting them in healing.

- Gather to hand everything you think you may need: the witness, crystals, sending device, pendulum, paper and pen for notes.

- Prepare your energies for healing as thoroughly as you would with the client present.

- Hold the witness or focus your gaze on it. Although you have obtained conscious permission you should also check whether you have Higher Self to Higher Self permission to proceed. Dowse or intuit the answer. If you get a feeling of 'No,' disconnect your energy, tidy things away and get on with your day. You can check back later as it may just be the wrong time. Repeated 'no' responses may indicate that it is not appropriate for you to do the healing and the client may be advised to ask for help elsewhere. If yes continue.

- Place the witness on the sending device. If you have several intuit the best one for the client.

- You may now choose which crystals are needed for the healing and arrange them as feels most appropriate. With a full body photo you can place crystals for individual chakras or the subtle bodies, put the individual in a crystal net or simply arrange the crystals as you intuitively feel they are needed. Remember 'less is more' may apply.

- Once you have chosen and placed the crystals dowse how long they need to remain in situ before you recheck them. It may only be minutes, it could be hours, or even days.

- If the layout is to be left for more than minutes ensure it is placed somewhere out of reach of fiddly fingers or animals.

- Now make your notes, file them, report back to your client and disconnect your energy until it is time to check the layout again.

- When you recheck the layout you may feel you need to change some stones or take the healing down. Remember to cleanse any crystals you remove in just the same way that you would after a healing with the client present.

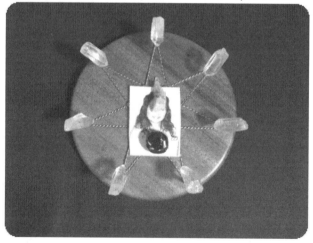

Distant healing is one way you can put yourself into healing. I used this layout to clarify my channelling of the 'still small voice within' using one of Steve's copper plates, a tiny phenacite crystal point coming into my crown chakra, a merlinite crystal on my brow and a covellite tumble on my heart chakra.

Chapter Thirteen:
Special Forms of Quartz

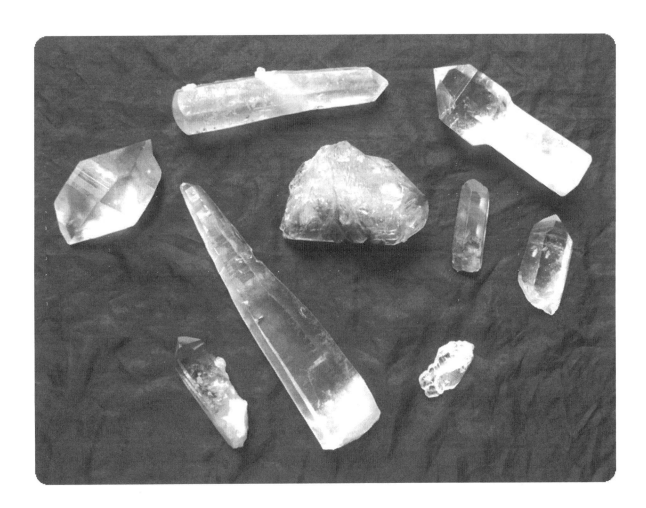

Special Forms of Quartz

Crystal healers have found that the formation of quartz crystals will affect the specific properties of the quartz. Certain forms have been named and categorised as 'master crystals' and have been ascribed metaphysical properties. Much of this has information been channelled by healers over the years. Whether you choose to work with quartz in this way or not it is helpful to know what other healers mean when using these terms and interesting to explore the different energies that come with different forms.

Generators

Generator crystals have six even natural facets which join together to form a terminated apex. Often they are cloudy at the bottom of the crystal becoming clearer towards the top. The more they are used the clearer and brighter they seem to become. Clear quartz generators are sometimes termed 'male' and are often used to channel energy, whereas milky quartz are sometimes termed 'female' and can be used to draw out stale energy.

Clusters

Clusters are groups of crystals which have grown together. They are helpful for positively energising communal environments.

Clusters, including beds of amethyst, may be used for charging other crystals. Don't place soft stones onto clusters as the quartz may scratch them.

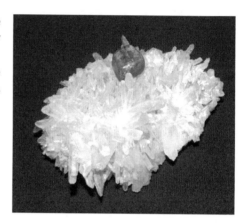

Etched Quartz and Record Keepers

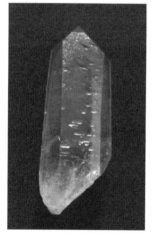

Some believe that the etched markings on these crystals are a form of Lemurian or Atlantean writing resembling cuneiform and that they have been imprinted with ancient wisdom. Record Keepers have at least one triangular marking on one of the six faces. They may be used as a focus in meditation to connect you to ancient wisdom. Simply running your fingers over the markings may uncover some of the information contained within.

Double Terminated Quartz (DTs)

These crystals have a natural termination at both ends of the crystal. The double termination enables them to direct energy inwards and outwards through either end of the crystal. Herkimer diamonds work in this way.

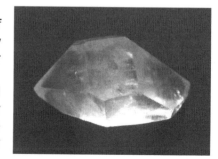

DTs are complete in themselves and exhibit well balanced energies. The DT can be placed above or on areas of energy blocks to help energy flow again. They are useful placed above the crown to open spiritual awareness and for clearing the energy of the spine.

Tabular Quartz (Tabby)

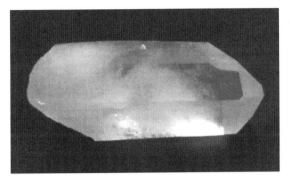

These crystals have a flattened shape with two of the opposing six sides being larger and wider than the others. The tabby has a very calming energy that can be comforting if someone is upset. Tabbies become like old friends and tend to get personalised to their user.

Phantom Crystals

Within some crystals can be seen smaller 'ghosts'. These markings demonstrate the growth pattern of the crystal, it will have stopped its growth and restarted when the conditions were right again.

These crystals are symbolic of the many phases of spiritual and personal development that can be experienced over a lifetime, and the refinement of the soul over many incarnations. Like the phantom crystal we have phases of rapid growth and times where nothing seems to be happening. These intervals are often necessary periods of rest and integration. A phantom crystal can help us develop patience on our spiritual journey. When the time is right we will move forwards again.

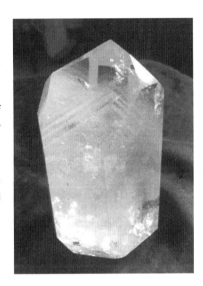

Barnacle Crystals

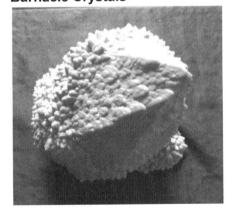

The surfaces of barnacle crystals are covered with smaller crystals. The central large crystal represents the 'wise old soul' and the smaller ones are attracted to it. These crystals can be used to symbolise the passing of knowledge between teacher and student, or between generations. They can also aid the emotions experienced when an older family member passes over and are particularly good used when meditating on group, community and family issues. These crystals are ideal to place in the classroom or workshop space.

Key Release Crystals

These are crystals which have an indentation in the shape of an inverse crystal. This is where another crystal has grown and then been released from the mother crystal.

The key release crystal is a good metaphor for motherhood, as such it is useful for parents learning to allow their children to grow into independence as young adults. It can also be used to meditate upon the nature of letting go gracefully.

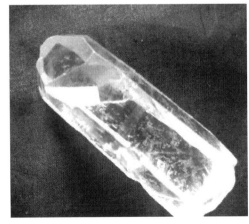

Elestials

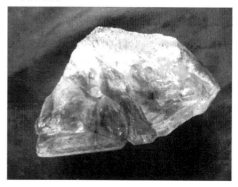

Elestials have terminations covering the body of the main crystal. This often gives the crystal a rugged or stepped appearance; they are also known as skeletal crystals. They are often smoky quartz.

These crystals are useful for making earth energy connections and can be powerful shamanic crystal allies. Elestials have a very high vibration and are believed to align the physical plane with angelic vibrations. As a meditation crystal they can heighten awareness of other realms.

Sceptre Quartz

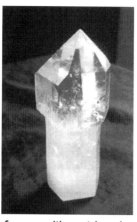

Here a larger crystal has formed around the stem of another crystal. Sceptres can be powerful and are useful for dealing with issues concerning the base and sacral chakras. They have a somewhat male energy!

Placed on your altar the sceptre quartz can be used to represent the Divine masculine.

Transmitter Quartz

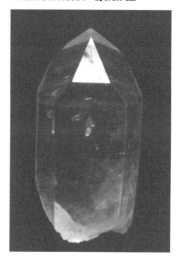

These crystals have two seven sided faces with a triangle between them. They aid connection with the Higher Self. Numerological interpretation of the number 7 indicates a search for hidden Truths and 3 is associated with clear expression. The 7-3-7 configuration can be seen as an ally in communicating with higher levels of consciousness and seeking spiritual insights.

Use the triangular face to gaze into, or hold it to your third eye. You can then ask for clarification and help in understanding an issue. For example what on the surface may look like a challenge or an unwanted event in our lives could reveal a deeper and more positive meaning when examined from a higher perspective.

Channelling Quartz

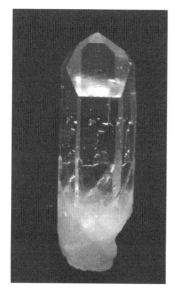

A channelling crystal has a large seven-sided face opposite a small triangular face. These crystals can be used for intuitive work and meditation. 7 is the metaphysical number symbolising the seeker of deeper Truths. 7 is also believed to be the number of qualities which human consciousness needs to attain to access and channel the wisdom of the soul. These qualities are: love, knowledge, freedom, manifestation, joy, peace and unity.

In meditation gaze into the larger 7 sided face or hold it to your brow.

Dow Crystal

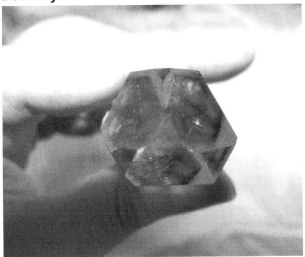

A Dow has the qualities of both a transmitter and a channelling crystal creating a beautifully balanced energy.

Dows have alternating seven sided and three sided facets and the faces are evenly proportioned. The Dow manifests a perfect geometry; the septagons indicate that we must first access our inner truth before we can manifest our divinity through the trinity of the triangular facets.

Use a Dow for channelling healing energy, or for meditation.

Laser Quartz

These crystals accelerate and focus the energy flowing through them. They have a long shape tapering towards a very small termination. They are precise and powerful tools which can be used to cut away heavy energy in the aura. Because they can cut into the aura like a surgeon's scalpel they must be used with care.

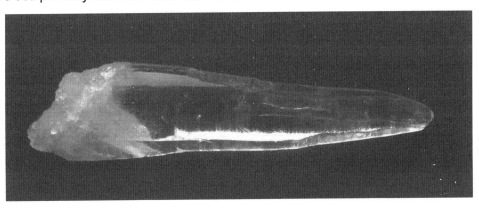

Tantric Twins

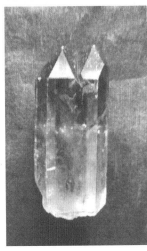

These crystals have grown harmoniously together side by side. They share a common base and have two distinct terminations. In a tantric twin crystal neither dominates.

These crystals are excellent for working on close relationships, particularly romantic, loving partnerships. They are symbolic of the need to be joined together, united by a common purpose, whilst retaining individuality and not being totally absorbed into the other.

Isis Crystals

The Isis crystal has a five-sided main face. Named after the Egyptian Goddess the Isis crystal is a feminine form of quartz which can help you connect with your inner Goddess.

The Isis supports the qualities of love, understanding and comfort. It makes a good ally for therapists as it supports a compassionate, receptive and empathic manner.

Placed upon your altar the Isis crystal can represent the Divine Feminine.

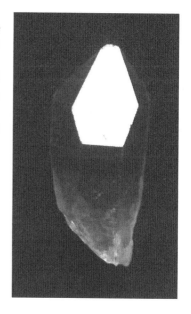

Bridge crystals

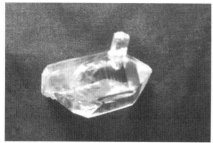

A bridge occurs when a smaller crystal penetrates a larger one and is partially in and partially out of it. The bridge can be used to connect where one party has wisdom to impart to the other, for example between Higher Self and self, or teacher and student.

Faden Crystals

Faden crystals are usually flattish in shape and can be identified by a fine white 'thread' running through them. One theory is that they are created when the Earth moves during earthquakes or during the slow movement of tectonic plates, breaking the crystals which then knit together again. Fadens are good for making connections, particularly repairing something that has been broken, whether that is a trust issue with someone, or a broken vow.

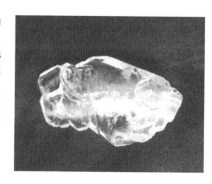

Time Link Crystals

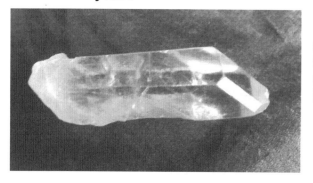

These crystals have a parallelogram on one of the main faces. They are used as bridges that the astral self can travel upon in order to consciously connect with other selves existing in other times and places.

Window Quartz

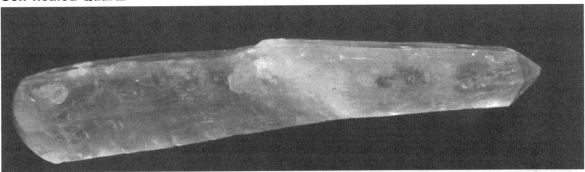

Window quartz crystals have an additional diamond shaped face between the body and the main facets. It is believed this crystal may help you find intuitive answers to questions, bypassing the ego or intellect. Windows are used for clarity and direction. If you are having problems and aren't sure why, a window crystal can be a useful ally to gaining personal insight. Pose your question and then gaze into the window with an open mind. Notice any words, images or inspirations. Sometimes answers arise later. Carry the crystal with you or put it under your pillow. Notice any guidance that comes through synchronicities or dreams.

Self-healed Quartz

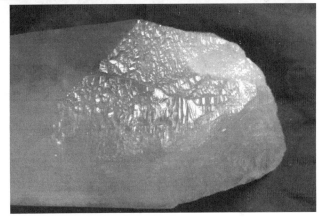

These quartz crystals have literally healed themselves as at some stage in their development they have been broken and knitted themselves back together. There may be a change to their angle or axis at the point of the break. They are good for physical repair in the body, especially assisting with bone knitting, though obviously broken bones should be properly set first so that they heal as straight as possible!

Another type of self healing occurs at the base of a crystal where it is broken away from the matrix and grows many tiny terminations at the broken end. These are lovely crystals to use for healing wounds, both physical and emotional.

Veil Crystals

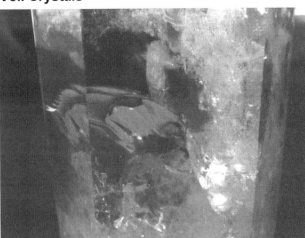

These crystals contain a veil like inclusions which float within the crystal. Beautiful shapes can often be discerned and these may give you insight into the nature of the crystal. This crystal contains ethereal wings.

Rainbow Crystals

Rainbows occur where light is diffused into its constituent colours. The rainbow is created through a fault within the crystal, showing us we don't have to be perfect to be beautiful. Rainbows are excellent allies for people who are experiencing sadness, loss, grief or depression.

Chapter Fourteen:
The Energy of the Space

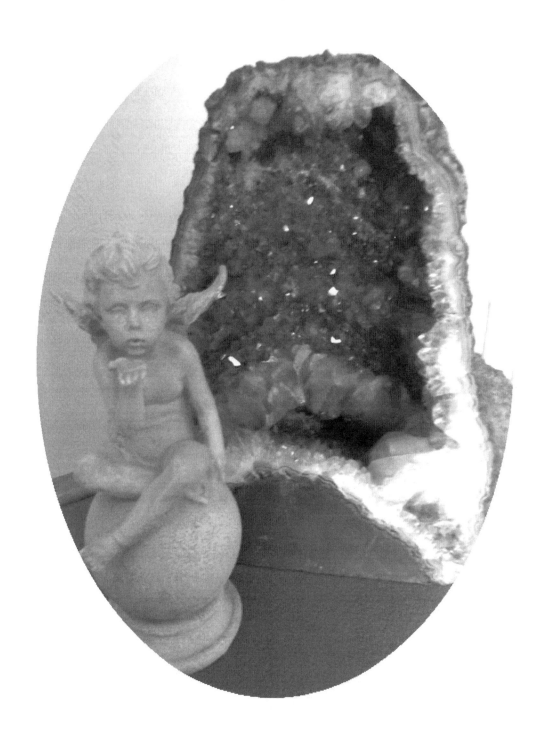

Space Clearing

I studied Space Clearing before I started to work with crystals. This background has given me the insight that the most effective healings are carried out in rooms that are energetically clean. Your clients will relax and let go more easily in a cleansed space where the energy is free flowing. General daily life can cause a build up of energy in a space, particularly if there is any friction between people or illness.

Sometimes when you do a healing the client will let go of a lot of heavy energy. That is terrific for them and they'll often say how much lighter they feel afterwards, but you may be left with a room that feels energetically heavy and it will need cleansing before any more healing is carried out there. This is one good reason to invest in a proper therapy couch that you can thoroughly cleanse, rather than use the sofa. It will also save you backache and look far more professional. I'd advise you *never* do crystal therapy on the bed you sleep on. Mattresses absorb energy easily and can be difficult to cleanse, which means you could be trying to relax in someone else's stale energy. If you don't have space or cash for a therapy couch then a yoga mat or thick blanket on the floor is an option. Floors can be mopped or vacuumed clean and blankets shaken out.

When space clearing a room pay particular attention to the corners which is where stagnant energy tends to collect. Many tribal cultures have round buildings as they believe evil dwells in the corners. I don't see this energy as evil, just of a lower vibration.

Using Sacred Smoke

Sacred smoke has been a traditional spiritual cleanser across many cultures. The most popular methods today are smudging, a Native American method using a smudge bundle of herbs such as white sage or sweetgrass, or incensing using various fragrant gums such as frankincense or myrrh. Be wary of using cleansing smoke if you have any respiratory issues or if you are pregnant. Some people don't like smoke in the air, so do not smudge or incense a treatment room just before a client arrives. It is a good method to use at the end of the day which then allows the air to clear overnight.

Smudging

Carefully light a smudge stick and hold it over a fireproof dish so that fragments don't fall and burn holes in the carpet or your clothes. You might want to add some dry sand to the bottom of the dish to help you put the stick out when you are finished. Waft the smoke around the space using your hands, or preferably a feather or feather fan. You can also smudge your own energy and if you have someone else available to smudge you then you can turn 90° at a time and have the smudge directed from head to foot all around you.

Californian white sage is our favourite smudging herb, but it is endangered, so please purchase from suppliers who stock sage from sustainably harvested sources.

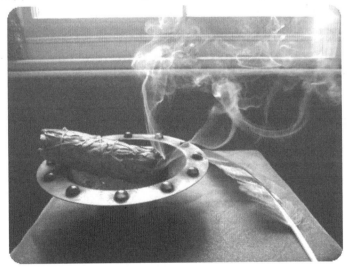

Solid Incense

The best incense to use for cleansing is solid incense which is made from natural gums and resins. You can buy charcoal disks which have a slight dish shape in the top especially designed for burning solid incense. Frankincense is one of the best spiritual cleansers, but there are lots of blends and mixes available. Opt for something that smells pleasant to you in the jar as although the smell changes when the incense being burned it will give you some indication.

When you light the charcoal ensure you have a fireproof dish or a censer to place it on and if that hasn't got a built in stand use something heat protective underneath such as a teapot stand as the dish will get very hot. Hold the charcoal disk firmly in tongs, not your fingers; I use old sugar tongs. Light the disk from the edge using a long match or a lighter. Let it sparkle all the way across and get hot before you add your incense grains.

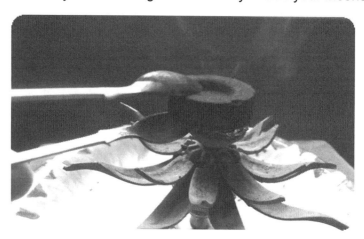

You can use your hands to waft the sacred smoke over your head and around your body. When you are cleansing a room make sure that the incense can burn without being a fire hazard and cannot be knocked over by pets or children. The charcoal stays hot long after the outside has turned to grey ash, so make sure it is fully out before you throw it away. If you need to leave the house you can let it burn out in a fireproof place such as a stainless steel sink or put it safely outside.

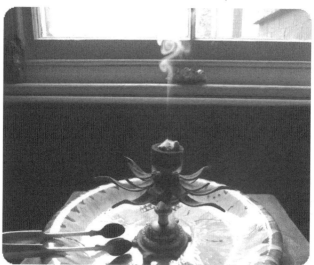

Stick and Cone Incense

Many joss sticks contain artificial perfumes that could pollute your atmosphere rather than cleanse it. If you burn stick or cone incense choose a variety which states clearly that it is made from all natural substances and ensure it makes you feel uplifted when you smell it. Nagchampa is a traditional incense which usually smells pleasant.

Fresh Air

Some modern buildings are so well insulated that there is simply not enough fresh air circulating. Toxins and heavy energies can build up as a result. Airing a room sounds old fashioned, but it is one of the quickest and most effective ways of bringing fresh energy in. I often open a window and air my healing room before and after a session. Make sure the room is warm enough for your client to relax in, use a heater and offer blankets if necessary.

Using Sound

Sound vibrations can break up and clear heavy energies. Most heavy energy is really just coagulated, dense, stuck or stagnant energy. Once it starts moving it lightens up and dissipates.

Tibetan Singing Bowls, Bells and Tingshas

Tibetan Singing Bowls are traditionally made of seven metals, although modern mass produced ones may not be. The energy radiates out from them into all the corners of a space. You play the bowl by holding it in one hand and rubbing a wooden mallet with gentle and even pressure around the rim. As well as cleansing your space the bowls can cleanse crystals and some therapists like to place the crystals they have used in the bowl itself and sound it. Only do this with robust tumble stones as the vibration can be too strong for more delicate crystals.

I'd advise you to find and buy your singing bowl in person from a store where the seller will let you try the bowl, as not all bowls will play for everyone. Your singing bowl should last you a lifetime, so see it as an investment. Never, ever, polish your bowl with metal polish, even if it looks dull. It may be ruined and not play again. You may wash it and dry it with a soft cloth if it is dirty.

Tibetan bells should always be supplied with a dorje. They are used in Tibetan Buddhism to represent the female and the male. You hold the bell in your left hand and the dorje in your right. They are powerful space clearing tools. You can either ring the bell with the clapper, or play it by stroking a wooden beater around the rim in a similar way to the singing bowl.

Tingshas are like small cymbals. You strike them gently together on the edge. They usually have a high sweet note and can add a blessing energy to your space. They also make a beautiful start to meditation. Follow the note into stillness.

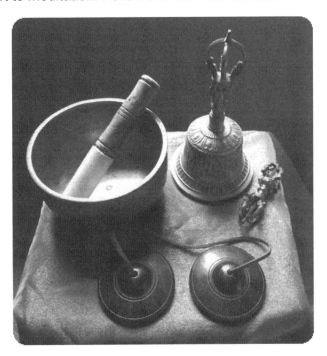

Crystal Singing Bowls

These bowls are made of reconstituted quartz crystal and are tuned to specific frequencies. They tend to be pricey so choose your bowl carefully. They are played in the same way as other singing bowls. Do not hit a crystal singing bowl with a mallet as they can be fragile and crack or chip. The sound from a crystal singing bowl can be extremely powerful and penetrating, therefore you will only need to play it for a minute or two. I love to light a tea light inside mine, creating a magical atmosphere in the room.

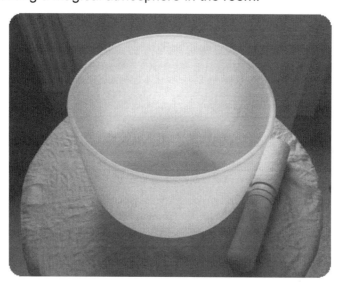

Gongs

Gongs can sound beautiful and are sound healing instruments in their own right. The best makes used by Sound Therapists are usually very expensive, however old dinner gongs and less well known makes can be much more affordable and are often resonant enough to clear the energy in a room.

Rattles

Rattles are usually cheap and cheerful and come in a wide variety of designs, you can even make a simple shaker for yourself using a small container and lentils. Again they work on the principle of breaking up stagnant energy with the sound vibration they make. You can shake them around your room to clear it paying particular attention to any areas where the rattle sounds dull or muffled.

Using Essences

Just as there are protective essences available on the market so there are cleansing formulas. Some sprays also contain floral waters which can be helpful for refreshing the energy of a room and for cleansing the aura. I find rosemary and juniper waters are helpful cleansers and provide a subtly fragrant base for adding the essence drops.

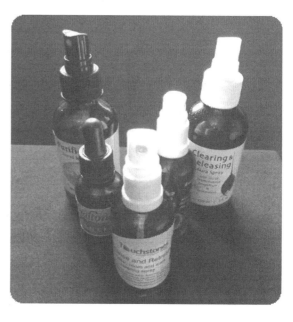

Be wary about using any essence sprays containing essential oils around people who may be contraindicated. Essential oils are potent substances and anyone who could be pregnant, has allergies, epilepsy, or is in delicate health should not be exposed to essential oils without first consulting a qualified aromatherapist.

Crystal Altars

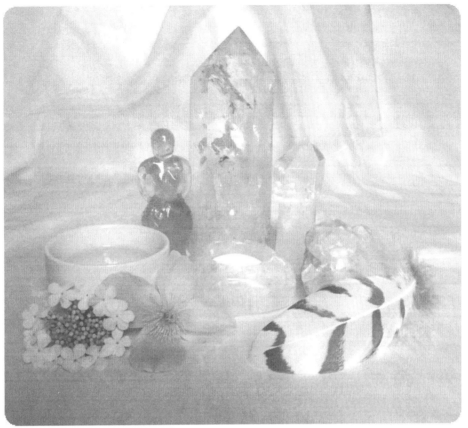

Whilst setting up a crystal altar is not an essential component of Crystal Therapy I find it brings a sense of the sacred to proceedings and helps me to feel centred and ready to do healing. My own crystal altar is semi-permanent and I only change the items on it when I feel the need. Refreshing the water and lighting the candle is part of my preparation for a healing.

The Elements

When you set up an altar you are welcoming all the Elements into your healing space. Use items to represent each Element. For example:

A feather represents Air
A lit candle represents Fire
A bowl of spring water represents Water
A crystal represents Earth
A symbol of the Divine represents Ether

The fifth element, Ether, is represented here by my amethyst Goddess sculpture and the sceptre quartz represents the God for balance between the Divine Feminine and Divine Masculine. Altars are very personal, you may prefer a statue or picture of Christ, Mother Mary, the Buddha, Kwan Yin, an angel, a favourite prayer, a sacred symbol, a guidance card, anything which strengthens your sense of Divine connection. You may also like to add something fresh from the natural world such as flowers.

Geopathic Stress

There are several types of Geopathic stress (GS). They can cause disruption to the energy field of most living organisms and prolonged exposure may to lead to serious illness. A number of other names are used to describe these phenomena including 'negative green'. 'Geopathic stress' is a term which covers all of the harmful Earth energies. I feel it is more important to discover the whereabouts of these lines than to categorise them.

Subterranean Water Veins

Subterranean running water, sometimes referred to as 'black streams', causes distortion of natural Earth energies. The water is usually deep underground, so you would not be aware of its presence. Because water is naturally variable the lines of stress caused by black streams may meander and can vary greatly in width. Surface water does not give rise to these problems.

Certain mineral concentrations, fault lines and underground cavities have a similar effect on Earth energies. The wavelength of natural Earth energy distorted in this way becomes harmful to most living organisms.

Hartmann Grid Lines and the Curry Grid

Hartmann Grid lines were discovered in 1950 by a German medical doctor, Ernst Hartmann. The lines form an electromagnetic grid around the Earth, running North to South and East to West, and extend vertically. The North to South lines appear approximately every 2 metres and the East to West lines appear approximately every 2.5 metres. According to Dr. Hartmann, the worst place that a person can sleep or work is over a 'Hartmann knot', where two Hartmann lines cross, as harmful radiation is intensified at this juncture.

The Curry Grid was discovered by Dr Manfred Curry and Dr Whitmann. These lines run diagonally North East to South West and South East to North West forming a diamond shaped grid. These lines are spaced around 3-4 metres apart depending on where you live. They have not been found to be very detrimental unless you are spending time over the intersection of two lines, termed a 'Curry crossing'.

The grid lines rise straight upwards, so for example everyone in a block of flats could be affected, even the people in the top flat. These lines are not normally very wide, usually less than 21cm, but they can get wider at full moon, during sunspot activity, or changing weather conditions.

Dowsers normally use dowsing rods to locate Geopathic stress. I also like to use a metal spiral pendulum which works well for me. Try both approaches and see what suits you best.

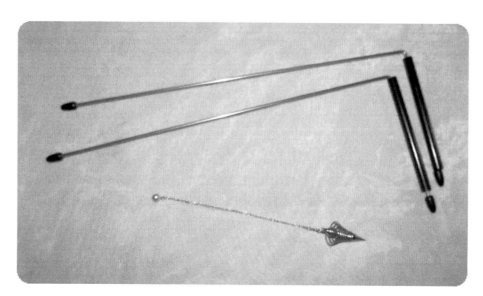

Geopathic Stress and Illness

Geopathic stress has been found to be a common factor in many serious and minor illnesses and psychological conditions, especially those conditions in which the immune system is compromised. German research has implicated GS in an increased risk of cancers forming. While GS may not be the direct cause of cancer, it is believed that it weakens the body and makes it more susceptible to cancer.

Other health problems which German researchers have claimed may be linked to GS include immune deficiency disorders, and chronic fatigue syndrome or ME. Some lesser effects which may be taken as possible early warning signs are chronic body pains, headaches, sudden signs of physical ageing and restless sleep. Some have also claimed it is a factor in cases of infertility and miscarriages, cot deaths, behavioural problems and neurological disabilities in children. GS is not generally accepted in the UK and unless more research in this area is carried out it is likely to be largely ignored as a possible causative factor in illness.

If you have a client who seems to respond well to your healing but doesn't sustain the benefits then it is possible that they are spending a lot of time in a Geopathically stressed location. You can dowse for how Geopathically stressed they are using the 1-15 dowsing chart provided in Chapter Four. A low number would suggest that GS is not a significant factor in their condition, a high number indicates that GS would merit further enquiry.

Physical Indicators of Geopathic Stress

The following are clues that there may be a strong level of GS in and around a home:

- Some organisms like geopathically stressed energy. These are called 'ray seekers'. Look out for infestations of slugs and snails, ants' nests and wasp nests. Bees are more productive when their hive is placed over GS. Mushrooms and medicinal herbs grow better over GS and oak trees like the energy but tend to grow twisted over it.
- Cats also like the feel of geopathic stress, but it isn't good for them. This may be why feline leukaemia and other feline cancers are so common. Dogs don't like it. Look at where a cat chooses to sleep and where a dog sleeps to help you assess a space. Of course cats also like comfort and warmth, so don't rule out all their favourite sleeping areas.
- Most mammals will sense GS and won't settle there if they can avoid it. Horses and cows stabled over GS may become sick.
- Many plants, especially fruit crops, will do very badly over GS. Stunted fruit trees which flower but don't fruit are a sign.

I came across GS as a young mother, before I'd discovered Crystal Healing. My house in Leicester had a line of ants' nests traceable from the street, through the front garden and out to the back garden. Snails were so numerous that it was hard to walk down the path after rain without stepping on them. One of our cats contracted feline leukaemia at a young age and died, shortly followed by cancer deaths in two of our older cats. We planted an apple tree, which flowered but never bore a single apple; the tree was aligned with the ants' nests. My baby daughter used to lie cramped up across the top of her cot widthways and I always wondered why she moved to such an uncomfortable looking position. Young children, like animals, are sensitive to GS and will move out of it if they can.

When I found out about GS and recognised the signs I installed a GS neutraliser indoors and I moved the cot. I moved the apple tree out of the GS line; it flourished and fruited from then on. It was visual, tangible 'proof' for me of the reality of GS.

I had more experience of GS when we moved to Wales. For the first couple of mornings in our new house my husband and I both woke with badly aching legs. I woke up exhausted, I felt like I'd aged overnight. At first I put it down to the exertion of moving, but then I realised that our pains would line up if we lay down side by side. I found the GS neutraliser in the packing boxes, plugged it in and from then on the aches and pains vanished and my vitality returned.

The questions below were written by Rolf Gordon and are from his book 'Are You Sleeping in a Safe Place?' Rolf has been a pioneer in the field of Geopathic stress in the UK. His book is a recommended read if you are concerned about GS. His website also has a lot of useful information.

> ### *How do I know if I'm Suffering from Geopathic Stress?*
>
> *If you cannot shake off an illness, depression or feel below par, ask yourself:*
>
> *1 Did my health problem begin shortly after moving into this home or place of work?*
>
> *2 Do I feel better when I am away from the home or place of work?*
>
> *3 Do any of my family feel uneasy about the 'atmosphere' at home?*
>
> *4 Did the previous occupants suffer from any serious or long term illness?*
>
> *5 Does the illness seem to be worse during autumn, or spring, or wet stormy weather? (underground water may be flowing at higher velocity)*
>
> *6 Were there any nearby disturbances, which may have caused underground water veins to flow into different channels under my house prior to my illness? (landslides, building and road works, working quarries and working mines etc)*
>
> *7 Does my home or any part of it feel unnaturally cold or damp?*

NB. In my experience some of these questions may indicate the presence of other phenomena, including energy portals or earthbound spirit activity, particularly questions 3 and 7. If these are the predominant characteristics you may be wiser to seek help from a specialist!

Geopathic Stress and Healing

GS may affect the quality of Crystal Healing that your clients receive. Dowse to check that your healing space is free of GS and check that lines do not cross where your client will be lying down.

You spend a good proportion of your life in bed. During sleep you are meant to rest and rejuvenate. However if you are exposed to GS during sleep, especially if you are sleeping over an intersection of GS lines, your brain and body may never receive the full rest they require to regenerate and heal. Make certain beds are not located over GS.

What Can You Do?

Move treatment couches, beds and favourite chairs away from GS lines. If someone has been ill you can dowse for a safer position for their bed or simply move the bed and see how the person feels in their new sleeping position after a few nights. As GS lines are usually narrow even moving the bed a small distance can make a big difference.

You can place smoky quartz crystal points at places where the GS energy enters and exits the home to change the vibration of the line. These will need frequent cleansing, charging and rechecking. Houseplants can also help to ameliorate the energy, but rotate them to rest them or they may get sick.

Professional Geomancers use a variety of techniques to move or neutralise the lines. I suggest approaching a specialist if you are concerned, or if your home has many of the signs and symptoms of GS then you may want to invest in a GS neutraliser as I did.

> ### Touchstones
> **Smoky Quartz:** Creates a more calming vibration along the GS line.
> **Lodestone**: Realigns the human energy field to the Earth's own energy field.

Sites of Power

Just as one place can make us prone to disease or depression, another can uplift us to a higher vibration, supporting our body and spirit. Such places have been sought after throughout history and held as sacred. Some are natural wonders like Ayers Rock, others are marked by prehistoric standing stones, henges, tors and earthworks and the building of shrines and temples. Some of these sacred sites have energies that are so powerful that it would be difficult to live on them full time, but they can raise our personal vibration when we visit them and can be good places to charge our crystals.

Alfred Watkins discovered that he could identify straight lines, which he called ley lines, in the landscape in the 1920s very close to where I live in the Welsh Borders. His book The Old Straight Track documents many such lines. Ley lines seem to connect significant numbers of sacred sites suggesting that early man was very aware of these energies.

Manmade Energies

We now live in a soup of different energies including artificial lighting, mobile phone masts, satellite broadcasts, wifi, microwaves and the vast array of electrical equipment that our ancestors didn't have to contend with.

Personally I feel we are human guinea pigs as this mix of different frequencies has never been experienced before. There is an urgent need for independent research into the bio-compatibility of manmade frequencies with natural background frequencies.

As far as I am aware researchers looking into mobile phone safety and phone mast safety, haven't assessed whether the energies emitted interfere with the human energy field. Even though science is aware that we have a 'bio-field' surrounding us the research seems to have been limited to whether devices directly affect the physical body when in use, for example whether mobile phones heat the brain.

We won't really know how our general health is being affected for several decades and the mix is so complex it is going to be difficult to sift through and work out which energies are causing problems. What is clear is that some people are more sensitive than others and find certain manmade frequencies uncomfortable.

I have noticed I develop migraine symptoms if I spend more than a couple of hours under fluorescent strip lighting. I would love to see these lights abolished in schools as studies have shown they affect concentration.

When I first met Steve he microwaved his food and thought I was odd because I didn't own a microwave. After living with me for a few years he visited a friend who put cold coffee back in the microwave in his shop to reheat. Immediately Steve had a sharp pain in his solar plexus. Thinking the microwave might be faulty the pair trooped up to the friend's flat where he had a brand new microwave. Exactly the same pain was experienced as soon as the microwave was switched on. Steve doesn't think I am quite so weird anymore!

The Schumann Resonance

First identified in 1952 by Professor Winfried Otto Schumann of Germany. These natural electromagnetic waves are the background energy of Planet Earth. They have a low frequency of about 3-60 Hertz, with a electromagnetic standing wave 7.83 Hertz. The fluctuations are thought to be caused by lightning in the Earth's atmosphere.

Some believe that the Schumann resonance acts like a 'tuning fork' for the mammalian brain as it seems no coincidence that the span of Schumann oscillations is very similar to that of brainwaves. Schumann wave simulators have been installed on NASA space flights for the health of the astronauts.

Modern living has made it virtually impossible to measure Schumann waves in cities as there are too many manmade electromagnetic signals. As technology progresses it becomes more difficult to find anywhere to live where the natural background energy of the Earth can be enjoyed without interference.

What Can You Do?

Although you cannot shield yourself from all the manmade frequencies being transmitted you can reduce your exposure to the technology which is under your control.

Electro Magnetic Fields (EMFs) get much weaker as you move away from them. The simplest solution is to move electrical items away from any sleeping and sitting areas so that they are out of the energy field.

Some devices such as mobile phones and laptops are designed to be used close up. You may choose to limit the time spent on these to reduce exposure. Try using the speaker phone rather than holding phones to your head and don't sit with a laptop directly on your lap. You can wear crystals to strengthen your own energy field or place an energy shielding crystal on your lap when making phone calls or using the computer. Crystals used around computers and electrical devices will need frequent cleansing and charging.

EMF meters have come down considerably in price and are an easy way of measuring the strength of EMFs emitted by electrical equipment. Seeing the needle move is good motivation for most people to take steps to limit their exposure!

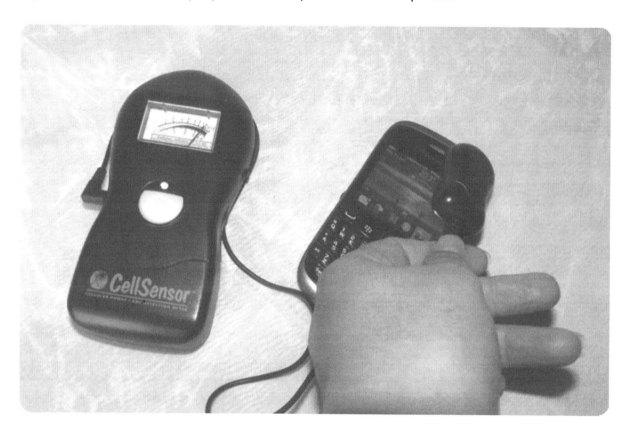

Touchstones
Smoky quartz: ameliorates the effects of EMFs.
Obsidian: creates a shield around the user which strengthens the energy field.
Lodestone: can restore the body's natural energy following exposure to EMFs.

Chapter Fifteen:
Advice for the Crystal Therapist

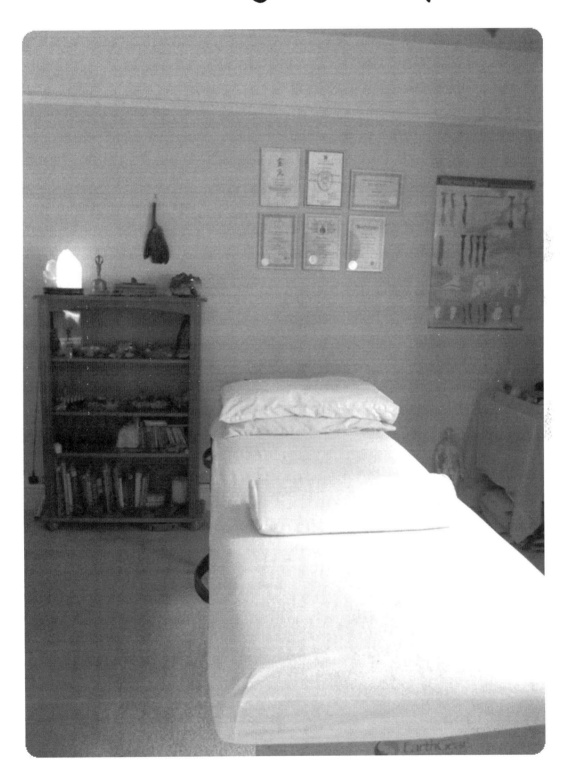

Raising Your Personal Vibration

As you progress on your healing path you will probably realise that you are changing. Your tastes in food, drink and lifestyle may alter and hopefully become healthier. You may move house, old friendships may fall away, your job may change, even your partner may need releasing! All of these things happened to me within the space of six years from starting to work with crystals and some would have happened sooner if I hadn't resisted them. They were all changes I needed to make and have been beneficial, though not without a level of emotional and physical upheaval at times.

Try not to fight change and instead recognise that this is a natural process. You are changing, therefore your external world will reflect this. Change happens in everyone's life anyway, whether desired or not. Commitment to a healing path with crystals may accelerate the pace of change. Problems occur when people try to 'put the brakes on' and keep life the same way it always has been. Try to relax and flow with your life. If you hold on tightly to things that are no longer in harmony with your highest good then you will hold yourself back.

Keeping your journal can help you through change. Try to keep a perspective and to take the longer view about what is happening. Sometimes short term discomfort is a necessary precursor to making long term improvements.

How far you take lifestyle changes is down to personal choice. You do not have to be a vegetarian, natural cloth wearing, fairtrade purchasing, defender of the environment to be a good healer, but then again you may be!

Touchstones

Pietersite: helps you to flow with the change, aptly nicknamed 'the storm stone'.
Labradorite: supports the exploration of new opportunities, an ally for transformation.
Mangano calcite: reminds you to treat yourself kindly through times of upheaval.

If you wish to consciously work on your personal and spiritual development you may want to consider the following:

Thought patterns

Are you a 'glass half full or glass half empty' person? It's better to maintain a hopeful mindset; you are much more likely to enjoy life. Check the quality of your conversations. How often do you indulge in gossip, criticism, or moaning sessions?

How do you feed your mind? What kind of television do you watch? Films? News? Positive news seems to be in short supply if you use the media as your guide. If you are a news addict you could start to view the world as a hostile and violent place. Remember news is selective and that the most horrific and dramatic events get top billing. Every day millions of heartwarming things happen, people are being kind, courageous, helpful and considerate. It isn't considered newsworthy. So are you watching or reading material that winds you up or drags you down? Could you swap for something more uplifting?

Are you a spiritual warrior or a spiritual worrier? Worry is a habit that drains your energy and diverts it from positive uses. Worrying about something rarely proves useful! If you have a problem write it down on paper, consider possible options and then take action, or talk it through with someone you trust for advice.

Being Present in the Now
Where is most of your energy? Is it wrapped up in the story of your past? Is it trying to run ahead of you in the future?

The past is history
The future a mystery
But today is a gift, that's why it is called the present.

This nugget of wisdom was taught by a colleague to all of her pupils when I was a school teacher. Really this moment is the only time we have, and the only time in which we can be useful, yet we spend so little time with our thoughts in the present. The point of power is in the Now!

Meditation
Meditation calms the mind and it can improve your intuition and ability to receive wisdom from your Higher Self. Even short periods of time spent meditating have been proven to reduce stress. Try to make space for at least five minutes of peaceful stillness each day, *especially* if you are busy and don't think you have the time!

Friendships and Relationships
Do your friends and relations support you? Are your conversations mostly positive? Is there a healthy balance of support or is it one-sided? It is wise to be aware of your boundaries. Helping a friend through a rough patch is fine as long as she'd be right there for you too! Some healers have a habit of compulsively helping others so they do not have to look inwards at their own issues.

As you change it is natural for some friendships and relationships to drop away and new ones to come in. Your energetic frequency is changing, so unless your friends or partners are also evolving in the same direction a gap will open up where you no longer resonate with each other. You may suddenly realise you have nothing much in common any more.

Jobs, Hobbies and Pastimes
Don't be surprised if what used to be an all consuming job fails to motivate you any more, or if an absorbing hobby no longer interests you. Let yourself flow with changes that occur and keep up to date with yourself. As one door closes another opens. Sometimes change will happen quickly and dramatically, sometimes more subtly, notice where your Spirit is guiding you.

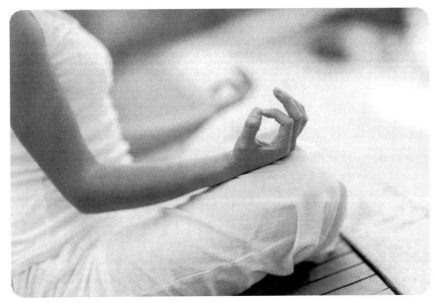

What is a Healing Crisis?

In an ideal world our clients would come along for a healing and feel wonderful immediately afterwards. Sometimes this is exactly what happens, however there is often a clearing out phase after healing which may feel quite unpleasant for a day or two. This detoxing is what is commonly termed a healing crisis.

An analogy that is sometimes used is to imagine a pond. The water may look fairly clear on the surface, but lots of junk has collected on the bottom of the pond and it is polluting the water. You want to have a good clear out so you start hauling out the old boots, bottles and cans, but as you do so the quality of the water muddies and the pond looks awful. You know that if you let the water settle back down it will clear itself naturally in a day or two and then it will be cleaner than before.

Crystal therapy sometimes hauls the 'old boots' from a client's energy system and in the process their energy gets stirred up and they can feel rather murky just like the pond water. It can take a few days for their energy to settle down again, during which time they may notice diverse symptoms which are due to the energetic detoxification process.

Here are some of possible symptoms of a healing crisis:
Feeling cold and shivery
Tearfulness
Belching
Loose and/or smelly bowel movements
Flatulence
More frequent need to urinate
Vomiting
Flu like symptoms
Feeling very tired
Generally feeling 'under the weather'

As you can see many of these symptoms are natural biological processes via which the body clears waste products or harmful substances from its system. Generally these are good signs that some unhelpful energy has indeed been shifted.

If discomfort is felt when the crystals are placed during the session then check whether it is okay for your client to stay with that feeling for a few minutes to see if it eases off. Often stones feel heavy at first and then become lighter after they have been in place for a few minutes. If your client would like you to move the stone then remove it and see if it feels appropriate to replace it with another stone with a more gentle action. If that doesn't feel right you can take the crystals off and ask your client to sit up and have a drink of water to settle them before you decide whether it feels right to proceed with the treatment.

Let clients know that if they suffer symptoms like those listed soon after their treatment then they are probably experiencing a healing crisis. They don't need to worry as these symptoms should improve by themselves within 24-48 hours, however if they are experiencing anything which causes them severe discomfort or anxiety, or if they suffer more prolonged symptoms, they should seek medical advice. It may be something unrelated to the healing. It wouldn't be very therapeutic to confuse the onset of appendicitis with a healing crisis for example!

After a healing clients are best advised to rest and relax as much as possible. If healing crisis symptoms arise they should stay warm and drink water to help flush the old energies out of their system. They may help the process along by taking a bath, perhaps with a handful of sea salt dissolved in it, or by taking a shower. Ask them to let you know what is happening and make a dated note in their records.

Releasing stuck and unhelpful energy can often be achieved more gently over time with minimal side effects for the client. I would never deliberately provoke a healing crisis, but sometimes a big shift happens and the body wants to release a problem all at once.

Occasionally someone gets up from my treatment couch feeling ice cold and shivery and I know that some very deep shifts in the core of their energy body have occurred. I'll give them a blanket to wrap around themselves, ground them well and allow some extra recovery time before they leave, plus offer a hot drink if they want one.

It is very normal for a client to need to use the bathroom immediately after a session as the flushing out can begin quickly. I take this as a good sign.

Some of my most memorable healings have had unpleasant after effects for a day or two afterwards. For example one lady wanted to get pregnant and had been trying with no success. After a healing she contacted me to tell me that she'd had such vile smelling flatulence the next day that she'd had to leave meetings to release it. She described the smell as, "The Devil's own." Later that month she became pregnant. I believe the congested and stagnant energy that had been stuck around her sacral chakra and womb area had been preventing pregnancy and moving these energies resulted in the need to release them quickly from her system. A case of short term embarrassment for long term gain!

It is hard to predict whether anyone will experience a healing crisis after their treatment so it is wise for clients to book appointments on days when they can rest and relax if necessary afterwards. Resting also allows the body to rebalance itself more effectively and to integrate any changes that have occurred during the healing.

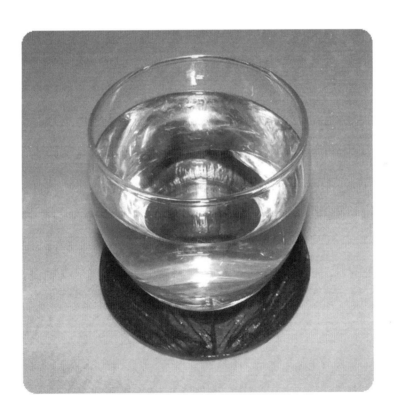

Maintaining Professional Boundaries

Be wary of making your clients into friends. You may get on very well with some of them, but your boundaries could get blurred if you start socialising or talking about your life in general. Clear boundaries are even more important if there is an attraction. Stop seeing the client professionally if this is the case. You must not have a romantic liaison with a client. You may recommend they see another therapist. Remember to detach energetically from your clients at the end of each healing session.

Keep your telephone boundaries clear. When is it appropriate for clients to contact you? Short calls, a text, or an email to report progress between visits are sometimes helpful, but ensure that you aren't being used to give free extra consultations. Consider getting an answering machine that allows you to screen your calls or use a mobile phone number for your work which you can switch off after a certain time, or at weekends.

Your energies can be drained by a phone call, which you have probably experienced if you've ever supported a needy friend or relative. Keep a small bowl of crystals by the phone and choose one to hold as energetic support when you have a needy caller.

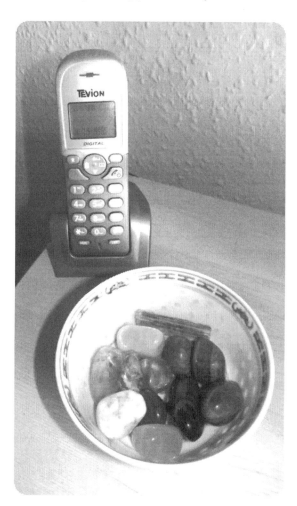

Touchstones

Kyanite: detaches energetic cords which form between people.
Obsidian: shields and strengthens the aura.
Key Release Quartz: releases people to make their own way in the world.

The Karpman Drama Triangle

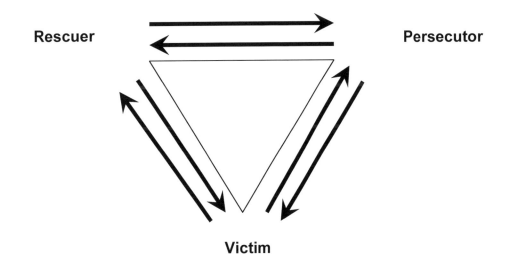

Rescuer   **Persecutor**

Victim

Psychologist Stephen Karpman described a common dynamic that occurs in relationships and which can apply to therapy situations. It is very easy for the client to fall into playing the Victim and the therapist to become their Rescuer. These roles are not healthy and they do not help a client move into their power and heal.

It is easy to slide between the roles, for example the Victim may bring out the Persecutor archetype in the therapist.

Signs that your therapist-client relationship may be unhealthy include:
- Offering your help unasked for (Rescuer)
- Allowing yourself to become the person that the client is dependent on (Rescuer)
- Enjoying the power or control you have over another's life (Persecutor)
- Not letting the client make their own choices (Persecutor)
- Client contacting you frequently between sessions (Victim)
- Client making unreasonable demands on your time (Victim)

If you take on the role of Rescuer and your client abuses your generous nature you will end up feeling like the Victim! Most therapists will fall into this trap at some point, so don't beat yourself up about it, renegotiate the boundaries, or extricate yourself as gracefully as you can and learn from the experience. Ultimately the answer to avoiding this unhealthy game is to own your power, to always aim to empower your clients and to set clear boundaries.

Should Healers Charge for Healing?

The question of whether healers should charge in return for giving healing is an ongoing debate. Here I present the arguments as I see them and my own view on this issue.

In the 'Healing Should be Free' camp the reasoning seems to run:

- Healing is a 'God given' gift; as such it would be wrong to take advantage of the gift and make money from it.
- Healers use Universal energy and that costs the healer nothing, therefore it would be unreasonable to put a price on it.
- Healing is a calling, not a profession.
- Many people cannot afford much and wouldn't come forward if healing were charged for.

In the 'Charge for Healing' camp the arguments run as follows:

- Charges represent the time and personal energy spent working with each client rather than the use of Universal healing energy. Clients are paying for the undivided attention, time and skills of the therapist over the duration of the therapy session.
- Clients often respond better when they have invested something into their treatment. They are more likely to respect the healer as a professional and so they are also more likely to listen to and follow after care advice.
- Healing should involve a fair exchange of energy, it shouldn't be a one way flow where the Healer just gives and the client just takes. Money can be viewed as energy, indeed it is called 'currency' and it represents the client's part of the exchange.
- Healers have to make a living just like anyone else. If they don't charge for their services then most would have to take a 'day job' that would impact on the number of people they could help.
- Healing is as valid a job as plumbing, hairdressing, or any other line of work. You wouldn't walk up to a hairdresser and demand a free haircut or call a plumber and get your leaky pipes fixed for free!
- The Healer will have invested in their training and they may also have had to purchase equipment and tools for their chosen modality. Asking for payment is therefore wholly reasonable as a return on this investment.
- Charges have to cover business overheads such as room hire, heating, lighting, practitioner insurance, registration with professional bodies, advertising, accountancy and consumables.

It isn't too difficult to see which side of the charging divide I stand on! If you have qualms charging as a newly qualified therapist you could offer lower introductory rates whilst you build your experience. Some therapists who do not need to earn an income from their therapy collect money for a chosen charity and state a suggested donation. My personal feeling is that you should receive some form of payment in exchange for your time, skills and energy.

Chapter Sixteen:
Crystallography

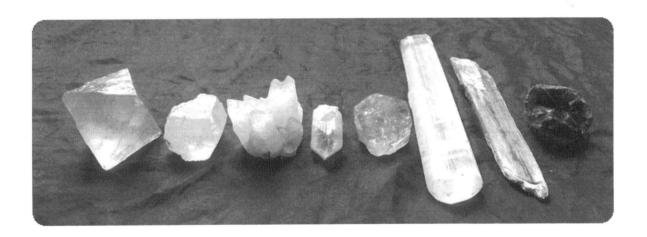

The Composition of the Earth

The Earth is structured in layers. We live on the very thin (relatively speaking) cooled layer called the Crust. This layer is floating on the Mantle, only 25-90 kilometres down, which is still extremely hot and quite soft in places. Minerals are brought up from the Mantle by volcanic processes. It is believed that the Inner Core of the planet is solid and mainly iron, with smaller amounts of nickel and other metals. The Earth's core is believed to be hotter than the surface of the Sun. The Outer Core is entirely molten.

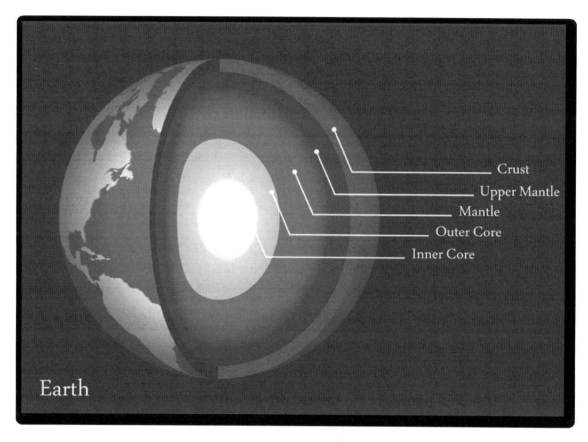

The Earth contains 92 elements which occur naturally, just eight of these form 98% of the weight of the Earth's Crust. The majority of the Crust, around three quarters by weight, is made up of oxygen and silicon, which is why the quartz family, silicon dioxide, are the most abundant. Most of the rest is composed of aluminium, iron, calcium, sodium, potassium and magnesium.

There are over 4000 known minerals in the Earth's Crust, but only 100 or so are common. A few, such as gold, copper and sulphur, are single elements, termed 'native' elements. The majority are chemical compounds made up of several elements.

Crystal Formation

Most minerals form from molten fluids that have risen towards the surface, cooled and solidified; in the cooling process crystallisation can occur. Crystallisation begins when the temperature of a liquid drops beneath its melting point. For water this is 0 degrees Centigrade, below which ice crystals will form. Rocks have far higher melting points, often over 1000 degrees C.

When cooling happens quickly, for example in lava flow from a volcanic eruption, the process is brief and only tiny crystals can form, pumice is a good example; it has cooled so quickly that many air bubbles are trapped within its structure. Sometimes the cooling is so sudden that there is no opportunity for crystallisation and glassy minerals, such as obsidian, with an amorphous structure are formed.

Crystals have highly organised internal structures and their atoms are arranged in a lattice pattern. When crystals have grown in a suitable environment the structure of their internal lattice may be seen reflected in their external shape, however the internal lattice structure of the same mineral will always be constant whether you are holding a perfect looking crystal or a rough chunk. Different factors can affect the growth of the crystal including temperature, pressure, available space and the presence of trace elements.

Crystals tend to form most perfectly in cavities and fissures in rocks because of the space available. Where space is restricted they may form as a solid mass; we refer to minerals with no external crystal form as massive. This is exemplified by the difference between rock quartz points and rose quartz. Rose quartz is usually found in massive form like the chunk on the right below. It rarely forms points and those formed are often tiny as you can see from the little cluster on the left.

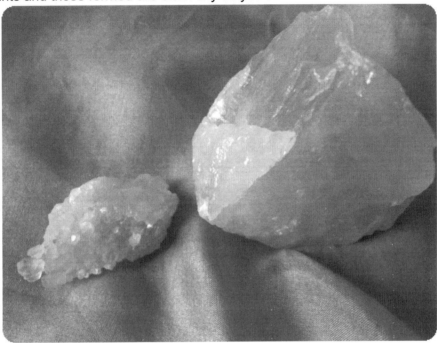

Time taken for crystallisation to occur varies immensely, from hours for example with ice crystals, to days in the case of salt crystals, to thousands, possibly millions, of years for larger crystals formed in slowly cooling metamorphic rock. As a generalisation the longer the time taken to crystallize the larger the crystal specimen that forms.

When examining your crystals it is worth using a magnifying glass or even a microscope. You will notice more this way. For example inclusions that look like brownish inclusions to the naked eye are revealed under magnification as golden cacoxenite crystals in this little amethyst.

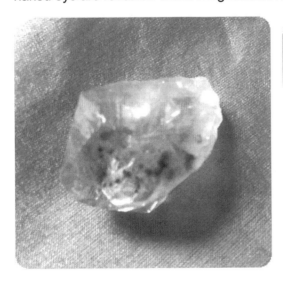
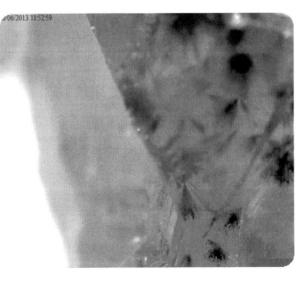

Cleavage

Crystals tend to break, or 'cleave', along the planes of their weakest atomic bonds. For example selenite will break most cleanly along its length following the striations. This 'sacrificial' piece of selenite was immersed in water for a short time for teaching purposes. The water loosened the bonds so much that it fell apart easily along its length.

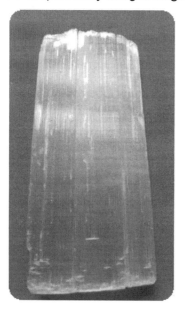 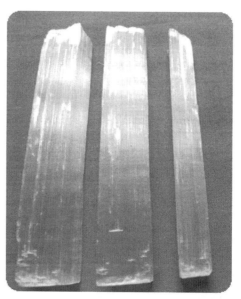

If you drop a calcite or celestite tumble and it breaks you will be left with a flat edge. Calcite will break into perfect rhomboids in this way and Is often available to purchase in this form.

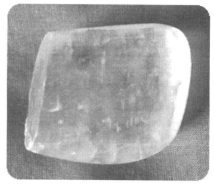

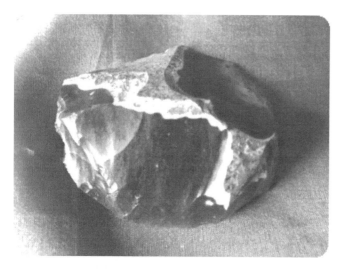

Some stones don't cleave cleanly like this. Quartz has a tendancy to fracture in a way which mineralogists call conchoidal, meaning 'shell-like'. This can leave very sharp edges, so be careful as they can cut skin. Our early ancestors exploited this to create cutting tools such as this flint scraper which has been patiently chipped at all around creating an edge which is still sharp thousands of years later.

Understanding the way a crystal cleaved used to be an important skill for gem cutters, which has now been largely superseded by advances in technology and diamond edged saws.

Hardness

Minerals each have a specific hardness. The accepted measure of hardness is called Mohs' Scale. It was developed in 1822 by German mineralogist Friedrich Mohs. Each mineral on Mohs' scale is capable of scratching the ones below it and will in turn be scratched by the ones above, so we move from the very soft to the very hard. If you go 'rock hounding' the Scale may help you identify your finds using everyday items such as coins and penknives.

1	Talc	Easily scratched by a fingernail
2	Gypsum	Scratched by a fingernail
3	Calcite	Scratched by a copper coin
4	Fluorite	Scratched easily by a pocket knife
5	Apatite	Barely scratched by a pocket knife
6	Orthoclase	Scratched by a steel file
7	Quartz	Scratches window glass
8	Topaz	Scratches glass easily
9	Corundum	Cuts glass
10	Diamond	Hardest known natural mineral, will scratch anything

The stones on the scale are an order of hardness, but they are not spaced evenly like the markings on a ruler, for example the gap between Corundum and Diamond in hardness is much larger than any of the others. A hardness of at least 7 is a good guide for jewellery. Anything softer should be worn with care for occasional use as it will scratch and dull over time.

Mohs' Scale is a reminder of why we should keep our crystals stored carefully and transport them with care; harder stones will scratch and chip softer ones if they are loosely rattling together and eventually the softer stones will look very sorry for themselves!

As a generalisation softer stones, such as sulphur, halite and malachite are excellent for absorbing unhelpful energies, whereas harder stones are good for directing or amplifying energy. Mineral Hardness Kits like mine are cheap to buy, but will not contain a diamond!

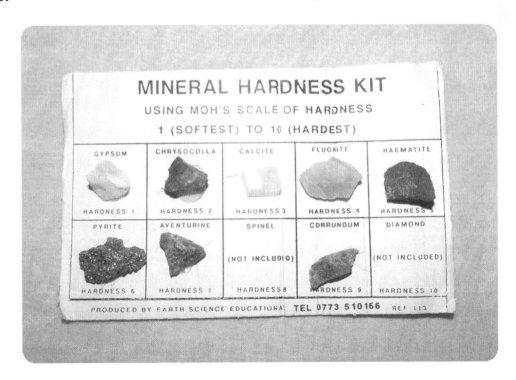

Gem Mining

As Crystal Therapists we have access to stones from all over the world. Although some crystals such as quartz are widespread, others are found in only one or two areas. Larimar for example is only found in the Dominican Republic. It would be an interesting exercise to find out where the stones in your collection are from and plot them on a World map.

Mining conditions worldwide are not always respectful of the workers or the local ecology. There are a few companies trying to deal in crystals under Fairtrade conditions, but these are the exceptions rather than the norm at present. Victoria Finlay's 'Buried Treasure: Travels through the Jewellery Box' gives you some insights into the lives of normal people involved in Gem mining around the world and I found it a fascinating read.

The most controversy surrounds the mining of diamonds. 'Blood diamonds' is a term used to describe those stones which are being mined in areas where there is conflict and then sold to fund war. These diamonds typically come from African countries where there is ongoing civil war. Not such a romantic image to link to an engagement ring! You can buy diamonds which are sold as ethical, traceable and conflict free.

In addition to the treatment of workers and communities mining can have serious ecological repercussions. Massive open pits have been excavated using heavy machinery to extract tonnes of diamond bearing rock. At the other extreme some diamonds are still being found by panning in river gravels, which is an ancient means of finding gemstones. It does muddy the waters and stir up the river bed so it isn't without consequences for wildlife, but it is a human scale operation rather than industrial scale one. Other stones commonly found using panning include rubies and sapphires in India.

The ancient methods of mining underground are still in use around the world for many gemstones, although the pick axe may have been swapped for drills and carts for trucks. Mining underground has always been potentially hazardous for the miners.

Without doing a lot of research it is hard to know how all of your stones were brought to the surface. Some healers prefer to work with British stones as you can be more certain that workers have not been exploited. The crystal below was purchased from a Rock and Gem show where a collector's crystals were on sale complete with provenance. This lovely smoky quartz came from the sandstones of the coal measures near Saundersfoot, Pembrokeshire. Knowing the pedigree of a crystal makes it extra special!

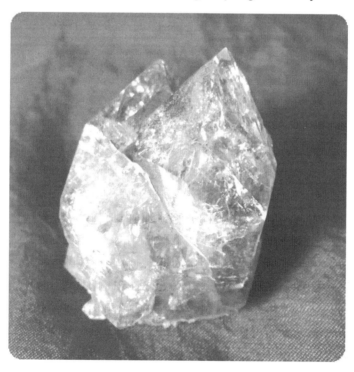

Chemical Formulae

Most minerals are combinations of elements, rather than native elements such as gold, copper or sulphur. Therefore the composition of the mineral can be expressed as a chemical formula.

As crystal therapists we can't be expected to memorise all of these, but awareness of the chemical constituents of your crystal can give you a clue to its properties and also how to store and handle it, so it makes sense to learn about the stones in your collection. For example lepidolite contains lithium which is used pharmaceutically to control mania and stabilize mood swings. Lepidolite is a very calming stone. Halite is salt and will dissolve in water. It even absorbs moisture from the air, so needs to be kept in dry conditions. Opal contains water in its structure. If it is kept in hot dry conditions it may lose its colour play.

The chemical formulae also show us crystals that are related to each other, which is interesting when looking at their shared properties. Most importantly you should be aware of minerals containing toxic elements; some are so poisonous they should not be used in treatments. There is no real need to use crystals with arsenic in their formulae for example. Please be cautious handling toxic crystals and *never* make gem waters or essences from these stones by the direct method. Poisonous crystals are often not labelled as such in shops and at fairs. Some crystal reference books give the chemical formula. Ensure you have at least one such book.

The table below shows the most common elemental symbols that you need to know to decode the chemical formulae of the majority of crystals. Toxic elements are highlighted in bold with an exclamation mark.

Element	Example crystal
Ag silver	silver Ag
Al aluminium	sapphire Al_2O_3 + Fe,Ti
As arsenic !	**realgar As_4S_4**
Au gold	gold Au
B boron	danburite $CaB_2Si_2O_8$
Be beryllium	emerald $Be_3Al_2Si_6O_{18}$
C carbon	jet C
Ca calcium	calcite $CaCO_3$
Cl chlorine	halite NaCl
Cr chromium	ruby $Al_2O_3(+Cr)$
Cu copper	malachite $Cu_2CO_3(OH)_2$
F fluorine	fluorite CaF_2
Fe iron	haematite Fe_2O_3
H hydrogen	opal SiO_2+H_2O
Hg mercury !	**cinnabar HgS !**
K potassium	amazonite $KAlSi_3O_8$
Li lithium	kunzite $LiAlSi_2O_6$
Mg magnesium	magnesite $MgCO3+Ca$, Fe, Mn
Mn manganese	rhodochrosite $MnCO_3$
Na sodium	sodalite $Na_4Al_3Si_3O_{12}Cl$
O oxygen	angelite $CaSO_4$
P phosphorus	apatite $Ca_5(PO_4)_3(F.Cl.OH)$
Pb lead !	**vanadanite $Pb_5(VO_4)_3Cl$**
S sulphur	sulphur S
Sb antimony !	**stibnite (Sb_2S_3)**
Si silicon	quartz SiO_2
Sr strontium	celestite $SrSO_4$
Ti titanium	rutilated quartz SiO_2+TiO_2
Zn zinc	zincite ZnO
Zr zirconium	zircon $ZrSiO_4$

Crystal Systems

Crystals can all be grouped into one of seven crystal systems. This is limited to seven because only seven geometric forms can fill a space without leaving gaps (tessellation). Crystal lattices are very neat and orderly! However different the crystals of a particular mineral may appear to the eye they will always belong to the same system. The geometric system the stone belongs to gives us some clues about its properties for healing.

Michael Gienger believed the human personality can be divided into the seven crystal types. This is a fun way to get to know the systems better and can be worth consideration therapeutically. Although Gienger suggested working with the crystal system which most closely matches your personality, I think there is mileage in working with the system which contains the properties you need to develop most in your persona at any given time.

The crystal personality types given here are summaries of the descriptions in Gienger's book 'Crystal Power, Crystal Healing'. See which structure describes yourself and those you know most closely. Gienger observed that people are naturally attracted to the crystals most aligned with their personality, so someone who has a cubic personality will tend to be drawn to cubic crystals. Take a look at the predominant crystals in your collection. What do they say about you?

The Cubic System

This is a system containing all crystals with a cube shaped inner structure. The most obvious actually form cubes, but this is a large system with more crystal shapes such octahedrons and dodecahedrons. These stones are practical and stable in nature. They may help with structural problems, such as skeletal complaints and repairs.

The cubic personality type is very organised and structured. They like set routines, plan their time carefully and think logically. They like the familiar; places, people, clothes and so on.

The biggest issue for this personality is their lack of flexibility. They don't like change or taking chances, or unforeseen events. They can depend too much on their rational mind and ignore intuition. They can cling stubbornly to routines and habits that are outmoded or no good for them.

Use cubic crystals when you need more order, structure, routine and stability in your life.

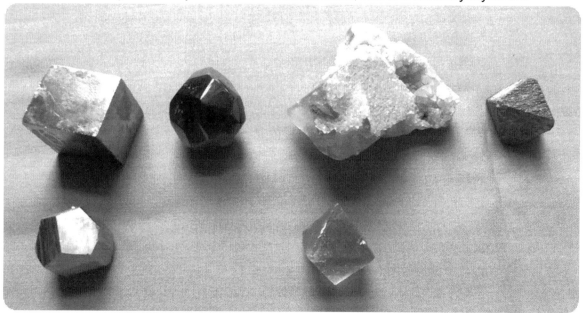

Touchstones

Iron pyrites: provides the energy to 'get on with it' and avoid procrastination.
Garnet: keeps you grounded and practical, supports energy levels.
Fluorite: promotes good organisation and self-discipline.
Lodestone: aligns the user with Earth's electromagnetic field.

The Hexagonal System

Many of the crystals in this system form hexagonal pillars. The Beryl family is hexagonal. These are good general healing stones. The hexagon has the smallest perimeter in relation to the enclosed area. The efficiency of this shape is utilised by honey bees for their honeycombs.

Hexagonal personalities are also 'busy bees'; efficient, hard working and motivated. They are clear thinkers with high standards. They can set their sights on a goal and work towards it effectively.

Hexagonal types don't like to be diverted or distracted and dislike time wasting. They usually care for their physical health, but illness can arise from overwork and too little relaxation. When ill they will often try to 'get back to normal' too quickly and make themselves worse. They can miss the richness of life because they are so focussed on their goals.

Use hexagonal crystals when you need to be more efficient and goal oriented.

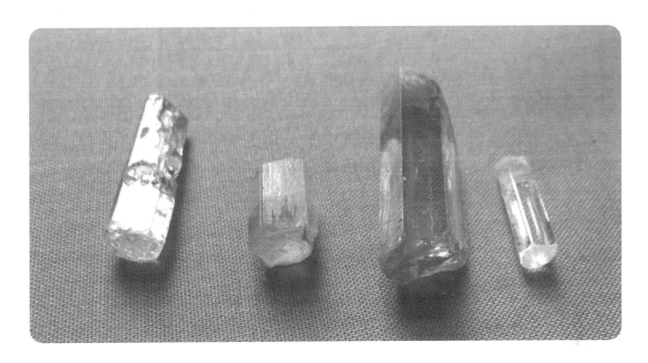

Touchstones
Aquamarine: calms agitated and difficult emotions and brings more peace and tranquillity.
Emerald: releases heartache and emotional wounds and supports an open, loving heart.
Heliodor: brings a touch of sunshine into the spirit to promote optimism and a 'can do' attitude.
Phenacite: connects one with the Divine aspect of Self.

The Trigonal System (sometimes considered by mineralogists as part of the Hexagonal System)

Comprises all crystals with a triangular inner structure including the quartz family. These crystals are very good at balancing subtle energies and stimulating energy flow. The triangle is the simplest geometric form.

The trigonal personality likes a simple, peaceful and uncomplicated lifestyle. They will try to do things in the easiest, most commonsense way and will put the least amount of effort in for the maximum results. They don't like to be rushed or pressured and are good at leaving their work behind them at the end of the day.

They can be somewhat lazy and so may take little exercise and become overweight and untoned. They dislike conflict and will avoid arguments, preferring to stay neutral. It is important for them to guard against being too inward looking and to maintain concern and feelings for others.

Use trigonal crystals when you want to release stress and attain a sense of peace, calm and simplicity.

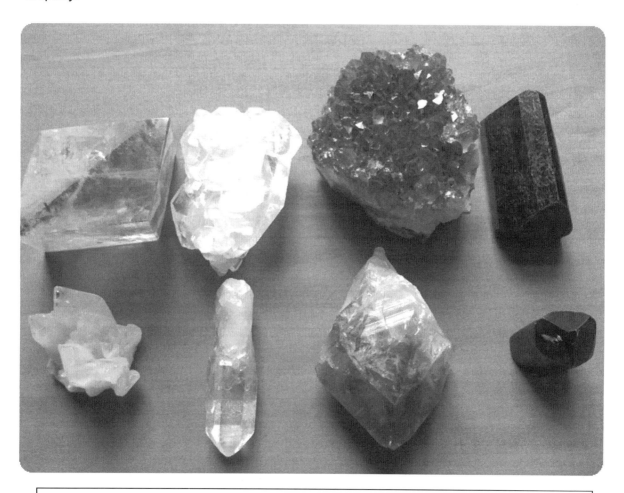

Touchstones
Calcite: soothes and gently heals, specific properties are affected by the colour.
Clear quartz: moves and directs energy, dubbed the 'universal healer' as it is so versatile.
Amethyst: spiritually uplifts, purifies and protects, a peaceful ally, supporting meditation.
Tourmaline: diverse range of energies, depending on type. Schorl grounds and protects.

The Tetragonal System

This system includes all crystals with a rectangular inner structure. They may grow as rectangular pillars, sometimes with pyramidal points. These crystals can absorb and transmute negativity.

Tetragonal personalities, like cubic ones, appear organised to the outside world, however they may be acting on the spur of the moment. They like to plan, but will adjust their plans whenever necessary and will drop or modify ideas and goals that aren't working out. Tetragonal personalities love the new and dislike routine and repetition. This gives them great scope for self development as they like a challenge, but others may see them as unpredictable.

This personality type can think clearly, but their thoughts are influenced by their emotions, so when their mood changes they may change their mind. Their appearance is a statement about themselves. They can lead a secretive 'double life' and this can produce feelings of guilt and shame. The challenge is for the inner self to match the outer self.

Use tetragonal crystals when you need to be more responsive and change your plans as you go along.

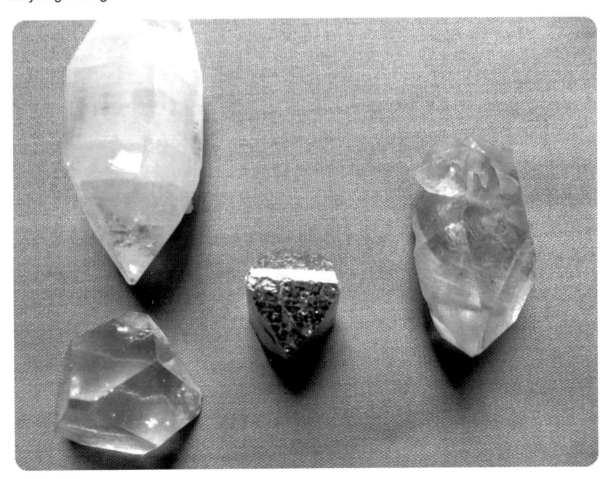

Touchstones

Apophyllite: spiritually uplifts and clarifies awareness of higher realms of being.

Zircon: supports a grounded spirituality that makes insights practical and of Earthly use.

Rutile: brings higher vibrations down to the physical level for rapid transformation of issues.

The Orthorhombic System

These crystals form around a rhombic inner structure and have a protective quality to them which enables the safe cleansing of old patterns.

The orthorhombic personality is normally well ordered and for long periods of time there can be great stability and little change. However when the orthorhombic personality has had enough, or loses interest in a routine or a situation they can change tack suddenly. Hence this personality type can change career, walk out of relationships, or move, with little or no warning. They quickly settle into their new lifestyle and life becomes very stable again, until the next time! They make good listeners and it makes them happy if others are happy.

Orthorhombic types may disregard their own wishes and needs for the sake of others, which over time can lead to one of the sudden changes of direction, or if their needs are suppressed may lead to depression.

Reach for orthorhombic crystals when you need the courage to make big life changes.

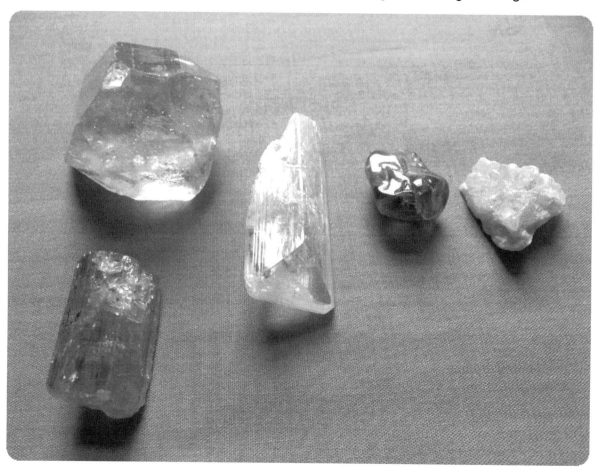

Touchstones

Topaz: Imperial topaz focuses the Will, blue topaz focuses the mind.
Danburite: encourages you to 'lighten up' and be aware of higher realms.
Peridot: protects and heals the heart, assisting loving transformation.
Sulphur: strongly cleanses and detoxifies, supports the right use of Will.

The Monoclinic System

These crystals have an inner shape of a parallelogram. They are directional stones which can clear obstructions in the energy field.

The monoclinic personality type is intuitive and spontaneous. They prefer flexible arrangements rather than concrete plans. Decisions are made from gut feeling rather than logic and so many people find this personality hard to understand and unpredictable. They need a peaceful, supportive environment to flourish.

This personality type can easily become overwhelmed with the demands of modern life and the way society is structured. Their self worth can be fragile and eroded by critical comments from others.

Use monoclinic crystals when you want to go with the flow, tap into your intuition and live more spontaneously.

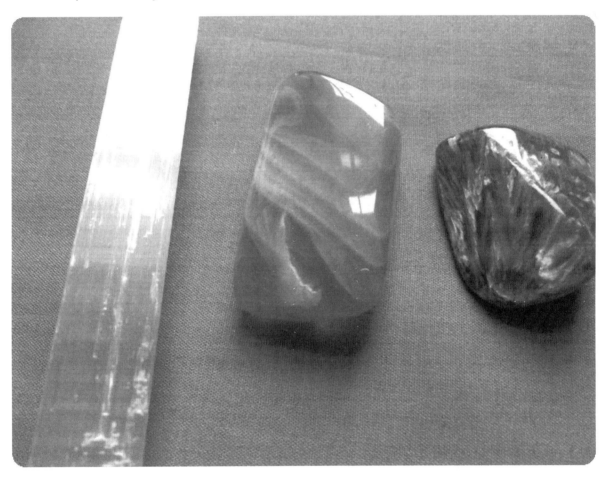

Touchstones

Selenite: purifies the energy field and transmutes heavy energies.
Moonstone: encourages harmony and acceptance of the cycles of life.
Seraphinite: supports and restores the healer's own energies.

The Triclinic System

These crystals have an inner structure in the shape of a trapezium. They can be used to access different states of consciousness.

When placed upright a trapezium is stable with a broad base, when turned upside down it becomes top-heavy and unstable. This personality type fluctuates between these two states and so potentially life can be erratic. Days may either go fantastically well or feel like an absolute trial from start to finish. Time either flies or drags. Life tends to be lived at one extreme or the other.

Some of these are classic Shaman stones. Use triclinic crystals when you need to be able to access an alternative viewpoint.

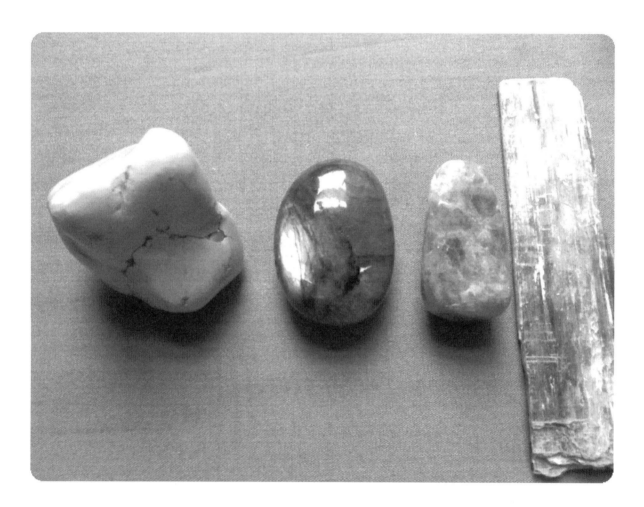

Touchstones

Turquoise: releases harsh judgements and supports a kinder, more forgiving viewpoint.
Labradorite: assists in navigating levels of reality, protecting our energetic boundaries.
Sunstone: carries a ray of optimism and vitality, promotes confidence.
Kyanite: releases restrictive ties formed in relationships, promotes harmony and unity.

Amorphous

Technically this is not a crystal system as this name means 'without shape' and is applied to stones with no inner crystalline structure. These stones remove rigid ways of thinking and promote self understanding.

The amorphous personality can live in the moment; everything seems fresh and new to them. They are spontaneous and grab new opportunities easily, letting go equally easily. In this respect they are childlike. They can be very creative, though usually have far more inspiration than they can manifest physically.

It is important that amorphous types retain their feeling of freedom and avoid feeling tied down as this can pull them out of living in the moment and make them miserable and apathetic.

Choose amorphous stones when you want to be more spontaneous.

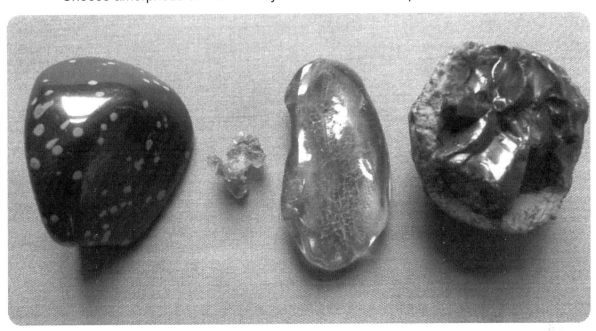

Touchstones

Obsidian: creates a field of protection around the user, deflects unhelpful energies.

Moldavite: activates awareness of Universal consciousness and raises personal vibration.

Amber: warms, comforts and emotionally soothes.

Opal: properties vary according to type, from calming blue opal to passionate fire opal.

Manmade and Man-altered stones

Nature has provided us with a vast array of beautiful crystals to work with. Some therapists choose to only work with natural crystals which have not been tumbled, polished or otherwise altered since they came out of the ground. Most crystal therapists also work with shaped, polished and tumbled stones as these are readily available, relatively affordable and generally more resilient.

Some stones have been treated more drastically. For example agates are dyed and sold in an array of lurid colours. Some therapists like to use them as these bright colours are less available in nature. I don't like dyed stones much and prefer to work with the palette Mother Nature supplies, but that is my personal choice and you can use them if you are drawn to them. As I understand it the 'crackle quartzes' have been heated up then quickly cooled to create the crackling inside and then dyed. Again I don't personally like this, but others find them appealing and some authors claim they have special metaphysical qualities because of this treatment. My personal feeling is the process shocks the crystals, but it is up to you to decide for yourself!

Citrine is most often 'burnt amethyst'; it started off life as an amethyst and was heated to change its colour to bright yellow. I prefer the feel of natural citrine which tends to be a pale yellow colour but is harder to obtain. Smokey quartz is commonly irradiated quartz, natural smokies tend to be lighter in colour, but it can be hard to tell the difference.

There are some stones that are often faked as the natural stone is expensive. One of the most commonly faked is Turquoise. White howlite is often dyed bright blue and is sometimes sold under the trade name Turquenite. Look out for trade names like this as they can be misleading.

In a different class are the quartzes which are treated with precious metals. I rather like these personally. I feel that something alchemical and magical happens when you bring these substances together. Aqua aura is quartz treated with gold vapour and it becomes an intriguing shade of blue. Ruby aura is quartz treated with gold and platinum creating shades from pinks to deeper reds. Angel aura is quartz bonded with platinum and silver creating iridescent shimmering colours reminiscent of a soap bubble.

Laboratories are capable of growing many precious stones these days and energetically I feel there is quite a difference between something that grew in the Earth and something created in a lab. The Siberian quartzes fall into this category. Sellers with any integrity will label things accurately, but there is a lot of unscrupulous dealing and the term 'buyer beware' applies, particularly when you are looking at expensive gemstones.

Natural obsidian is great to work with, but you will also come across manmade glass such as 'blue obsidian'. The market has a lot of glass being sold under misleading names such as cherry quartz, or goldstone which is glass and copper glitter. These are often pretty and may have colour healing properties, but they are not natural stones. Retailers often don't know the difference.

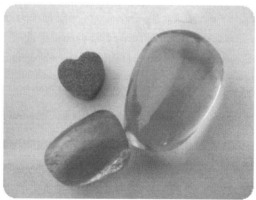

Appendix B is a list that Sue Lilly drew up with contributions from myself and others to help people navigate the minefield of treated stones and trade names.

Appendix A: The ACHO Stones

If you are studying an ACHO course then you will be expected to familiarise yourself with and make an in depth study of the following list of stones:

Clear quartz

Rose quartz

Amethyst

Smoky quartz

Citrine

Herkimer diamond

Other members of the Quartz family for example Carnelian, Jasper

The Beryl family including: Emerald, Aquamarine

Calcite

Tourmaline

Haematite

Pyrite

Fluorite

Garnet

This is not an exhaustive list of the stones you may use as a Crystal Therapist.

Malachite

Moonstone

Turquoise

Lapis lazuli

Obsidian

Labradorite

Celestite

Amber

Within the Touchstones Diploma course we also work with:

Ruby

Kyanite

Selenite

Appendix B: List to Clarify Stone Names and Types of Crystals
compiled by Sue Lilly, reproduced with kind permission

Usual name	Mineralogical name	Chemical Formula	More info
Agnitite	Quartz	SiO_2	TM name for quartz with Haematite from Madagascar
Amegreen	Quartz	SiO_2	Trade name for chevron amethyst and prasiolite from Africa
Ammolite	Aragonite	$CaSO_4$	Opalescent aragonite from Alberta, Canada
Amorite	Chalcedony	SiO_2	Trade name for druzy chalcedony from Mexico
Anandalite	Quartz	SiO_2	Trade name for druzy quartz with titanium from India
Angel Aura	Quartz	SiO_2	Trade name for quartz, lab-enhanced with platinum and silver particles
Angelinite	Quartz	SiO_2	TM name for white or milky quartz
Angelite	Calcium Sulphate	$CaSO_4$	Also known as blue anhydrite
Anyolite	Zoisite	$Ca_2Al_3(SiO_4)(Si_2O_7)O(OH)$	Common name for ruby and zoisite with tschermakite from Tanzania
Apache Tear	Obsidian	SiO_2	Translucent variety of obsidian (a volcanic glass)
Aphrodite	Colbaltoan Calcite	$CaCoCO_3$	Trade name for cobalto-calcite. spherocobaltite
Aqua Aura	Quartz	SiO_2	Trade name for quartz, lab-enhanced with gold particles
Aquatine	Calcite	$CaCO_3$	Blue-green calcite
Ascensionite	Basalt & dolomite	$(Mg,\underline{Ca})CO_3$	TM name for Basalt/dolomite/quartz from South Africa
Astaraline	Quartz, muscovite, cronstedtite	SiO_2	TM name for muscovite, cronstedtite, quartz
Atlantisite	Stitchtite & Serpentine	$Mg_6Cr_2CO_3(OH)_{16}\cdot4H_2O$ $((Mg, Fe)_3Si_2O_5(OH)_4$	Trade name
Auralite 123	Amethyst	SiO_2	Trade name for chevron amethyst with inclusions from Ontario, Canada
Austrian Crystal *			Glass with lead added to create extra sparkle.
Avalonite	Chalcedony	SiO_2	Blue chalcedony
Avalonite	Zoisite	$Ca_2Al_3Si_3O_{12}(OH)$	Trademark name for banded pale orange zoisite. Found in Washington State, USA
Azeztulite	Quartz	SiO_2	TM name for quartz with lots of bubbles/fractures
Balas Ruby	Spinel (red)	$MgAl_2O_4$	
Bixbite	Beryl (red)	$Be_3Al_2(SiO_3)_6$	Many colours of beryl are given specific names
Black Amber	Lignite	C_4	Also known as Jet
Black Hills Ruby	Garnet (pyrope)	$Mg_3Al_2(SiO_4)_3$	Type of garnet
Black Labradorite	Larvikite	Igneous rock	
Black Moonstone			Misnomer for diopside or even labradorite
Blizzard Stone	Gabbro		Trade name for gabbro (feldspar/mica/quartz/pyroxene)
Blue Goldstone *	Man-made glass		Trade name for a blue, glittery man-made glass aka nightstone or sandstone
Blue Obsidian *			Usually a man-made glass often from volcanic ash

Blue Storm	Agate	SiO_2	From Namibia
Boji Stone	Limonite	$FeO(OH) \cdot nH_2O$	TM name for pyrite, limonite, marcasite concretions from Kansas, USA
Bolivianite	Quartz	Sio_2	Ametrine
Burnt Amethyst	Quartz	SiO_2	Citrine
Champagne Aura	Quartz	SiO_2	Trade name for quartz, lab-enhanced with gold and indium
Cherry Quartz	Man-made glass		Red man-made glass
Chiastolite	andalusite	Al_2SiO_5	Aka Andalusite
Circle Stone	Flint	SiO_2	TM name for flint from Wiltshire, England
Clinochlore	Clinochlore	$Mg,Fe)_3(Si,Al)_4O_{10}(OH)_2 \cdot (Mg,Fe)_3(OH)_6$	Aka seraphinte
Coracalcite	Calcite	$CaCo_3$	TM name for golden calcite from Florida, USA
Cordierite	Cordierite	$(Mg,Fe)_2Al_4Si_5O18$	Aka Iolite
Crab Fire Agate	Agate	SiO_2	Aka Spiderweb carnelian (enhanced)
Crackle Quartz	Quartz	SiO_2	Lab treated quartz, often coloured
Crimson Cuprite	Chrysocolla and cuprite		TM name for chrysocolla and cuprite from Mexico
Crow's Coal	Carbon	C_4	Anthracite (coal)
Desert Rose	Gypsum	$CaSO_4$	Variety of selenite
Desirite	Quartz	SiO_2	Trade name for crystals containing phantoms
Dianite	Potassicrichterite	$K((Ca,Sr)Na)(Mg_5)Si_8)O_{22}(OH)_2$	Often mistakenly described as 'blue jade' or 'blue jadeite'
Dolphin Stone	Pectolite	$NaCa_2Si_3O_8(OH)$	Aka larimar
Dravite	Tourmaline	$NaMg_3Al_6(BO_3)_3Si_6O_{18}(OH)_4$	Brown tourmaline
Dream Quartz	Quartz	SiO_2	Trade name for quartz with epidote
Eilat Stone	Chrysocolla, malachite, azurite		Chrysocolla, malachite, azurite sometimes diopstase
Elbaite	Tourmaline	$Na(LiAl)_3Al_6Si_6O_{18}(BO_3)_3(OH)_4$	Mineralogical name given to a type of tourmaline (occurs in most colours)
Fairy Cross	Staurolite	$Fe_2Al_9Si_4O_{22}(OH)_2$	Trade name for staurolite
Fairy Stone	Calcite	$CaCo3$	Trade name for concentric calcite concretions from Quebec
Flame Aura	Quartz	SiO_2	Trade name for lab-enhanced quartz with titanium and niobium
Gaia Stone *			A glass said to be made with Mt St Helen's ash
Galaxite	Labradorite		Microcrystalline labradorite
Girasol	Quartz	SiO_2	Trade name for opalised quartz
Goldstone *	Man-made glass		Trade name for a orange/brown, glittery man-made glass aka sandstone
Goshenite	Beryl	$Be_3Al_2(SiO_3)_6$	A clear variety of beryl
Grand Canyon Wonderstone	Jasper	SiO_2	Banded jasper found in the Grand Canyon area of Arizona
Guardianite	Agerine, feldspar, riebeckite etc		Trade Mark name for a combination of agerine, feldspar and riebeckite
Gwindel Quartz	Quartz	SiO_2	Quartz with a twisted structure - see http://www.quartzpage.de/gwindel.html
Harlequin Quartz	Quartz	SiO_2	Quartz with lepidochrosite and/or haematite inclusions
Healer's Gold	Pyrite & magnetite	$FeS,$	Trade mark name for pyrite & magnetite from Arizona

Heliodor	Beryl	$Be_3Al_2(SiO_3)_6$	Name for golden/yellow beryl
Heliotrope	Jasper	SiO_2	A name for bloodstone
Herkimer Diamond	Quartz	SiO_2	Trade name for a double-terminated quartz from New York
Hiddenite	Spodumene	$LiAl(SiO_3)_2$	Green kunzite/spodumene
Ice Quartz	Quartz	SiO_2	Trade name for growth-interupted quartz from India
Icelandic Spar	Calcite	$CaCO_3$	Name for a clear variety of calcite, often orthorhombic crystals
Idocrase	Complex silicate		Also known as Vesuvianite
Indicolite	Tourmaline	$Na(LiAl)_3Al_6Si_6O_{18}(BO_3)_3(OH)_4$	Name for blue tourmaline
Infinite or Infinity stone	Serpentine	$((Mg, Fe)_3Si_2O_5(OH)_4)$	Trade name for serpentine from Africa
Lemon Chrysoprase	Nickeleon magnesite	MgCO3 with nickel	Name given to nickeleon magnesite aka Citron
Lemurian Aquatine	Calcite	$CaCO_3$	Trade name for blue-green calcite from Argentina
Lemurian Infinite	See Infinity Stone)		
Lemurian Quartz	Quartz	SiO_2	Trade name given to quartz points with fine lines and other markings on the side of the crystal
Lilac Lepidolite	Lepidolite	$(KLi_2Al(Al,Si)_3O_{10}(F,OH)_2$	Trade mark name for lepidolite from Africa
Lodestone	Iron Oxide	$Fe2+Fe_2^{3+}O4$	A variety of magnetite
Luvulite/Lavulite	Sugilite	$KNa_2(Fe,Mn,Al)_2Li_3Si_{12}O_{30}$	Trade name for high grade sugilite
Master Shamanite or Shamanite	Calcite	$CaCO_3$	Trade mark name for black calcite
Melody Stone	Quartz with many inclusions	SiO_2	Trade name a combination stone consisting of Quartz, Smokey Quartz, Amethyst, Cacoxenite, Goethite, Lepidocrosite, and Rutile
Merlinite	Chalcedony	SiO_2	Trade name for dendritic opal/chalcedony
Metamorphosis Quartz	Quartz	SiO_2	See Girosol
Mexican Onyx	Calcite/Marble	$CaCO_3$	Misnomer for banded calcite/marble
Moqui Marble	Limonite	$FeO(OH)\cdot nH_2O$	Trade name for limonite aggregates from Utah
Morganite	Beryl	$Be_3Al_2(SiO_3)_6$	Pink beryl
Mystic Merlinite	Gabbro		Indigo gabbro from Madagascar
Nebula Stone	Jasper	SiO_2	Aka Kambaba jasper
Mystic Topaz	Topaz	$Al_2SiO_4(F,OH)_2$	Topaz coated with a fine layer to create colour
Neptunite	Neptunite	$KNa2Li(Fe^2+, Mn^{2+})_2Ti_2Si_8O_{24}$	
New Jade	Serpentine	$((Mg, Fe)_3Si_2O_5(OH)_4)$	Misnomer for bowenite a variety of serpentine
Nirvana Quartz	Quartz	SiO_2	See Ice Quartz
Novaculite	Quartz	SiO_2	A form of flint from Arkansas
Opal Aura	Quartz	SiO_2	Trade name for quartz, lab-enhanced with platinum and silver particles
Opalite *	Man-made glass		Trade name for a man-made glass resembling moonstone

Erratum: Nebula stone and kambaba jasper are two different stones. They look like black and green photographic negatives of each other. Nebula stone has green dots and Kambaba jasper has black dots.

Ouro Verde	Quartz	SiO_2	Irradiated quartz
Pariba tourmaline	Tourmaline	$Na(LiAl)_3Al_6Si_6O_{18}(BO_3)_3(OH)_4$	Blue and pink tourmaline
Peacock Ore	Chalcopyrite	$CuFeS$	Trade name for oxidised chalcopyrite
Pecos Diamond	Quartz	SiO_2	Misnomer for a variety of double-terminated quartz from New Mexico
Picasso Stone	Jasper	SiO_2	A variety of jasper
Pink Lazurine *			Trade name for a manufactured, lab-grown pink quartz
Prasolite/Prasiolite	Quartz	SiO_2	Also known as green amethyst
Protector Quartz	Quartz	SiO_2	Trade name for quartz with haematite inclusions
Quantum Quattro	Shattuckite, chrysocolla, dioptase, malachite, smoky quartz		Trade name for a combination of shattuckite, chrysocolla, dioptase, malachite and smoky quartz
Que Sera	Quartz	SiO_2	Trade name for quartz and feldspar with inclusions from Brazil
Rainbow Aura	Quartz	SiO_2	Trade name for lab-enhanced quartz with titanium and niobium
Rainbow Moonstone	Plagioclase feldspar	$(Ca,Na)(Si,Al)_4O_8$	A misnomer/synonym for white labradorite
Reiki Stone			Apophyllite
Rosophia	Feldspar, quartz and biotite		Trademarked name for a combination of feldspar, quartz and biotite
Royal Azur/Royal Azel	Sugilite	$KNa_2(Fe,Mn,Al)_2Li_3 Si_{12}O_{30}$	See Luvulite
Rubellite	Tourmaline	$Na(LiAl)_3Al_6Si_6O_{18}(BO_3)_3(OH)_4$	Red or pink tourmaline
Ruby Aura	Quartz	SiO_2	a trade name for a type of quartz, lab-enhanced with gold and silver particles.
Satin Spar	Selenite	$CaSO_4$	Another name for selenite
Shaman Stone	Quartz	SiO_2	Trade name for quartz with inclusions Of chlorite, lepidochrosite and/or iron.
Shaman Stone (alternative)	Limonite	$FeO(OH)\cdot nH_2O$	See Moqui Marble
Shantilite	Agate	SiO_2	Trademark name for a banded agate
Sharylite	Alabaster	$CaSO_4$	Trade name for alabaster
Schorl	Tourmaline	$NaFe_2+_3 Al_6(BO_3)_3Si_6O_{18}(OH)_4$	Black tourmaline
Siberian Quartz *			Trade name for a manufactured, lab-grown quartz – various colours
Siberite	Tourmaline	$Na(LiAl)_3Al_6Si_6O_{18}(BO_3)_3(OH)_4$	Violet or purple tourmaline
Smoky Topaz	Quartz	SiO_2	Misnomer for smoky quartz
Sonora Sunrise		$(Cu,Al)_2H_2Si_2O_5(OH)_4 \cdot nH_2O$ & Cu_2O	Trade name for a combination of chrysocolla and cuprite from Mexico
Super Seven or Sacred Seven			See Melody Stone
Tangerine Aura	Quartz	SiO_2	Trade name for quartz, lab-enhanced with gold and copper particles.
Tanzan or Tanzine Aura	Quartz	SiO_2	Trade name for quartz, lab-enhanced with gold and indium particles

Tarnowitzite	Aragonite	$CaCO_3$	Aragonite (lead-rich)
Tempest Stone	Pietersite	SiO_2	Also known as Pietersite (Pietersite is a chalcedony)
Tiffany Stone	Fluorite	CaF_2	A name for opalised fluorite
Transvaal Jade	Grossular Garnet	$Ca_3Al_2(SiO_4)_3$	A misnomer for hydrogrossular green garnet
Verdite	Tourmaline	$Na(LiAl)_3Al_6Si_6O_{18}(BO_3)_3(OH)_4$	Green tourmaline
Victorite	Quartz	SiO_2	Trademark name for quartz with spinel
Water Sapphire	Cordierite	$(Mg,Fe)_2Al_4Si_5O18$	A misnomer/trade name for iolite/cordierite
Witches Fingers	Quartz	SiO_2	Quartz with various inclusions from Zambia
White turquoise	Howlite	$(Ca_2B_5SiO_9(OH)_5)$	A misnomer for Howlite
Youngite	Quartz	SiO_2	Brecciated jasper and drusy quartz
Z stone	Gypsum	$CaSO_4$	Trade name for concretions from the Sahara Desert

- Glass is a super-cooled liquid and is not crystalline. There are natural glasses – like obsidian. Many are man-made. All glasses are chemically SiO_2

Further Study

There are dozens of excellent books that I haven't listed here, so this list is by no means exhaustive or meant to be restrictive. Most of the books and videos listed are collected together for ease of purchase on the Touchstones Shop on my site. Links to websites are given in good faith, but I cannot guarantee every web page will be accurate or appropriate.

Crystals

You will need a selection of crystal reference books. No single book covers all the crystals in use. The Book of Stones is my favourite crystal tome. The Lilly's handbook is neat, portable and has the technical information you'll require. The Crystal Ally Cards are the ones I use throughout the Diploma course and with my clients.

The Book of Stones	Robert Simmons and Naisha Ahsian
The Crystal Ally Cards	Naisha Ahsian
The Essential Crystal Handbook	Sue and Simon Lilly

Energy Safety

The Psychic Protection Handbook	Caitlin Matthews

The Chakra System

Anodea Judith's DVD is an excellent introduction which bears watching several times. The Caroline Myss DVD is a live recording of a lecture she gave in the 90s, but other than references to the year 2000 it is as relevant as ever:

Wheels of Life	Anodea Judith
The Illuminated Chakras (DVD)	Anodea Judith
The Chakra System (Audio CD set)	Anodea Judith
Anatomy of the Spirit	Caroline Myss
The Energetics of Healing (DVD)	Caroline Myss

The Human Energy Field

Cyndi Dale's book is well illustrated and encyclopaedic in scope. Barbara Ann Brennan's book is regarded as the classic reference book for healers.

The Subtle Body	Cyndi Dale
Hands of Light	Barbara Ann Brennan

Crystal Nets

The Lillys have published several books of their crystal nets. I suggest you start your exploration with their original book of nets:

Crystal Doorways	Sue and Simon Lilly

Quantum Physics

Quantum physics is complex. I think the easiest way in is the DVD which presents key concepts for the layman. My advice is to buy the original drama documentary film not the extended edition, which is less accessible.

What the Bleep do we Know (DVD)

Vibrational Medicine	Richard Gerber
The Field	Lynne McTaggart

Traditional Chinese Medicine and the Meridians

Gienger's book is the only one I am aware of written specifically for Crystal Therapy. For a detailed set of charts with point location descriptions I use Sue Hix's publication. Between Heaven and Earth gives more insight into Traditional Chinese Medicine.

Healing Stones for the Vital Organs   Michael Gienger and Wolfgang Maier

Fourteen Classical Meridian Charts   Sue Hix

Between Heaven and Earth   Harriet Beinfield and Efrem Korngold
A free online version of their Five Elements Questionnaire: www.longevity-center.com

Healing on the Spine

Louise Hay includes a chiropractic chart of correspondences for the spine in her book. I use the wall chart by John Cross Clinics which can be ordered from his site.

Heal Your Body   Louise Hay

The Holistic Spine (A1 poster)   John Cross
www.johncrossclinics.com

Space Clearing

Karen's book was the doorway through which I entered the world of energy work and Denise Linn's writing has also been inspirational for me. Both authors utilise a form of Feng Shui which aligns everything to the front door. I prefer the traditional compass directions given in this manual. Choose one system or the other, don't mix and match.

Creating Sacred Space with Feng Shui   Karen Kingston

Sacred Space   Denise Linn

Electromagnetic Fields

The Powerwatch Handbook   Alasdair and Jean Philips
The Powerwatch site has more information: www.powerwatch.org.uk

Geopathic Stress

Are You Sleeping in a Safe Place?   Rolf Gordon
Rolf's site has more information: www.rolfgordon.co.uk

Ley Lines

Watkins' book is the classic text on ley lines.

The Old Straight Track   Alfred Watkins

Crystallography

Gienger's book has more information on crystallography than most. The DK Visual Guide is not about crystal healing, but great for technical information and photography. Its previous incarnation as 'Rock and Gem' was bigger in format and is worth seeking out. Victoria's book is well written account of her adventures as she travels the world finding out where gemstones come from. It appears to be out of print, but second hand copies may be found.

Crystal Power, Crystal Healing   Michael Gienger

Rocks and Minerals,   Ronald Bonewitz
the Definitive Visual Guide (DK)

Buried Treasure: Travels through the Jewellery Box   Victoria Finlay

All photographs and illustrations Author's own apart from:

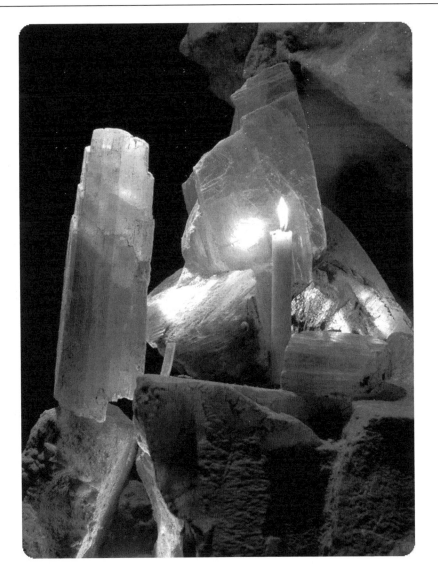

About the Author

Lauren D'Silva BA (Jt Hons), PGCE, Principal TSCT

Lauren is an experienced healer, teacher and writer offering crystal therapy, colour therapy, gem essences, channelled healing and spiritual guidance. A fully qualified teacher with twenty five years of teaching experience Lauren has taught Crystal Therapy to Diploma level for over a decade. Lauren caters for all levels of experience and expertise in her teaching, providing for the complete novice right up to those who have already completed their therapy qualification and are looking for continuing professional development.

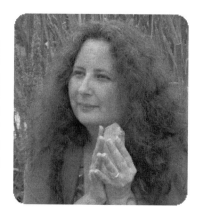

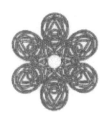

Lauren is Principal of Touchstones School of Crystal Therapy. The School provides professional training for Crystal Therapists. In addition to the ACHO accredited Certificate and Diploma courses the School also provides a Home Study Course and Continuing Professional Development (CPD).
Email courses@touchstones-therapies.co.uk
www.crystal-therapy.co.uk

The Affiliation of Crystal Healing Organizations

ACHO is the largest organisation for Crystal Therapy schools in the UK and was founded in 1988. All ACHO member schools have agreed to cover a core curriculum within their courses and to uphold the ACHO Training Standards. Providing you qualify with an ACHO school you can apply for a listing on the ACHO Practitioner Register. At time of publication Lauren is the Chair of ACHO.
www.acho.co.uk

Touchstones Therapies

Lauren offers Crystal Therapy, Colour Therapy, Hypnosis and Channelled Healing from her Practice in Mid Wales. If you live too far away to attend in person she can also work with you via Skype wherever you live in the World. Lauren specialises in spiritual development, past lives and cord releasing. If you would like to work with Lauren please contact her.
Email lauren@touchstones-therapies.co.uk
www.touchstones-therapies.co.uk

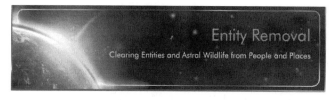

Lauren's husband, Steve Deeks-D'Silva is a Shaman specialising in the removal of stubborn, persistent and unhelpful energies. If you feel in need of his assistance please email a brief summary of the issue and a recent photo of yourself via email and he will give you a free initial consultation and a quote for any work required. Please note he does not offer telephone consultations.
Email steve@entity-removal.co.uk
www.entity-removal.co.uk

Made in the USA
Middletown, DE
30 April 2015